LIVING WELL WITH PERSISTENT PAIN

Living Well with Persistent Pain is a straightforward guide to understanding the challenges facing those who live with persistent pain.

This book offers valuable, easy-to-navigate guidance, answering key questions for everyone whose life is touched by persistent pain. Questions include: 'What is it like to live with persistent pain?'; 'Why is it so hard to explain persistent pain to someone else?'; 'What has psychology got to do with persistent pain?'; and 'Is it true that laughter and swearing can help with pain?'. This book shows how hard it is for the individual to self-manage in isolation, shares the evidence base for core psychological interventions, and highlights the role we all have to play in supporting those living with persistent pain.

Written by an academic expert health psychologist who also has NHS experience of working with people living with persistent pain, this book shares the evidence base in an accessible way. The accessibility makes it indispensable for anyone who wants to understand more about the role they can play in reducing the challenges faced by those living with persistent pain, whether they be the person with pain, their friends, family, employer, or health professionals.

Karen Rodham is a health psychologist and academic working at the University of Chichester (situated on the south coast of the UK). She specialises in researching how best to support those who live with complex and chronic physical health conditions, and has in the past worked in the NHS supporting people to live well with persistent pain.

BPS ASK THE EXPERTS IN PSYCHOLOGY SERIES
British Psychological Society

Routledge, in partnership with the British Psychological Society (BPS), is pleased to present BPS Ask the Experts, a new popular science series that addresses key issues and answers the burning questions. Drawing on the expertise of established psychologists, every book in the series provides authoritative and straightforward guidance on pressing topics that matter to real people in their everyday lives.

All books in the BPS Ask the Experts series are written for the reader with no prior knowledge or experience. For answers to everything you ever wanted to know about issues important to you, ask the expert!

Understanding Climate Anxiety
Geoffrey Beattie

Living Well with Parkinson's
A Guide to a Fulfilling Life
Angeliki Bogosian

Living with Grief
A Compassionate Companion
Sara Mathews

How to Eat Well at Every Age
Jane Ogden

How to FUEL your Resilience
A Practical Guide to Developing Resilience Skills for Professionals
Rose Aghdami

Living Well with Persistent Pain
Karen Rodham

For more information about this series, please visit: BPS Ask The Experts in Psychology Series - Book Series - Routledge & CRC Press

LIVING WELL WITH PERSISTENT PAIN

KAREN RODHAM

Routledge
Taylor & Francis Group
LONDON AND NEW YORK

Designed cover image: Getty images

First published 2027
by Routledge
4 Park Square, Milton Park, Abingdon, Oxon OX14 4RN

and by Routledge
605 Third Avenue, New York, NY 10158

Routledge is an imprint of the Taylor & Francis Group, an informa business

British Library Cataloguing-in-Publication Data
A catalogue record for this book is available from the British Library

Library of Congress Cataloging-in-Publication Data
Names: Rodham, Karen, 1970- author
Title: Living well with persistent pain / Karen Rodham.
Description: Abingdon, Oxon ; New York, NY : Routledge, 2027. | Series: Ask the experts in psychology series | Includes bibliographical references and index.
Identifiers: LCCN 2026019667 (print) | LCCN 2026019668 (ebook) | ISBN 9781041093985 hardback | ISBN 9781003649854 paperback | ISBN 9781003649854 ebook
Subjects: LCSH: Chronic pain | Chronic pain--Psychological aspects | Chronic pain--Patients | LCGFT: FAQs
Classification: LCC RB127.5.C48 R63 2027 (print) | LCC RB127.5.C48 (ebook)
LC record available at https://lccn.loc.gov/2026019667
LC ebook record available at https://lccn.loc.gov/2026019668

ISBN: 978-1-041-09398-5 (hbk)
ISBN: 978-1-041-09397-8 (pbk)
ISBN: 978-1-003-64985-4 (ebk)

DOI: 10.4324/9781003649854

Typeset in Joanna MT Std and Poppins, as briefed for the headers
by KnowledgeWorks Global Ltd.

To Gwen, Gerry, Leo, and the
other Gadds, the Richmonds, the
McCaheartys, the Hilarys and the Coles
whose siren call led me home.

CONTENTS

PREFACE

WHO IS KAREN RODHAM, AND WHY HAS SHE WRITTEN A BOOK ABOUT LIVING WITH PERSISTENT PAIN?

According to the British Pain Society, almost half of us in the United Kingdom will experience persistent pain (also known as chronic pain). Through this book I will share information that I hope will help you gain a deeper understanding of the challenges of living with persistent pain.

It is not my intention to tell people who live with pain what they probably already know. Instead, what I want to do through this book is raise awareness of the things that we as friends, carers, health professionals, employers, and other fellow human beings can do that will make it easier for those who live with persistent pain to live well in spite of their pain.

I want to bring to your attention some of the challenges that face those who live with persistent pain. I will share quotes drawn from my own and others' research and practice experiences that highlight what is called the 'lived experiences' of people with persistent pain. In other words, I will be sharing the stories told by those living with persistent pain. Through their generous sharing of their experiences, we can begin to see the world through their eyes and gain glimpses of what living with persistent pain might look and feel like. We can begin to think about our potential role in adding positivity instead of accidentally making things more challenging. If I have done my job well, this book will be a source of valuable information, tips, and practical tools for those who love, live with, care for, and work alongside people living with persistent pain.

But before we get started, I would like to introduce myself. I know that whenever I come across a book like this, my first thoughts about the author are 'Who are you?' and 'Why should I listen to what you have to say?'. So, in this preface, I want to tell you a bit about me. I hope that once you have read this, you will feel you know me a little better and be willing to hear (read) the things I want to share with you.

WHO IS KAREN RODHAM?

Hmmmm. How can I tell you about myself? When we meet people for the first time we tend to ask them what they 'do' for a living. I've always felt a bit uncomfortable with this, because what someone does is not necessarily a reflection of who they are. Maybe more useful questions could be: 'What's the most interesting thing you've learned recently?', or 'What is the first thing you want to know about someone when you meet them?', or 'What makes you laugh?', 'What makes you happy outside work?'. Inevitably though, when I am meeting someone new, I often fall back on the 'What do you do?' question. So here is my answer to that question and I'll answer the others too.

What do you do?

Right now as I write this, I am an academic working at the University of Chichester, based on the south coast of England. There are three key things that I think academics do:

1. **We teach**. We teach our students to question, to think critically, to make up their own minds after reviewing evidence. We teach them the value of learning. Most importantly, we are steadfast in our belief in our students' abilities and their potential (especially at the times when they cannot see it for themselves) and we help them to learn that they can do more than they believe possible.

Graduation is my favourite time of the year. It is a privilege to play a small part in the journeys of our students. They are the future of our profession and I am excited to see how they will contribute to it.

2. **We mentor**. We offer support to our students and help them learn how to navigate life as well as their studies, so they leave us with lots of life, study, and work skills that set them up for their futures. We help them to build their own confidence and competence so that they can go on and make a positive contribution to our world.
3. **We research and write**. We do our own research so we can contribute to our respective areas of expertise. We share our work, often in academic journals but also in more accessible formats. Maybe we will record a short video to share our findings. Maybe we will write for the local paper. Maybe we will give talks to local, national, and international meetings. Sometimes, we are able to write books. Writing books is one of the favourite parts of my job. I love having the opportunity to share the things I have learned, things that I think are interesting, useful, and hopefully helpful with as many people as possible.

What's the most interesting thing you have learned recently?

I never made the connection between the name *mange tout* (also known as a 'snow pea') and how we eat them. I know a tiny bit of French and know that *mange* means 'eat' and *tout* means 'all'. But I never put the words together. I heard someone on the radio explain that the name *mange tout* is essentially telling you how to eat this vegetable. You can pop it in your mouth whole and eat it all. *Mange tout!* Thinking about that experience again as I write, I can see that it is a useful example for what I want to do with this book. I am sure that some of what I share here will be familiar to you, but perhaps some of what I share may give you your own 'Aha!' moments as you realise you knew something at one level, but now you can see it and understand it more deeply.

What is the first thing you want to know about someone when you meet them?

The first thing I want to know when I meet someone is are they really present with me in that moment. It is not that I want lots of attention, but I do want to know that whoever I am talking with is fully listening to what I say. If we are not both present, how will we connect? I do not care who they are or what they do. I simply want to know that they are open to connecting and present at that moment.

What makes you laugh?

In the spirit of being my authentic self, while also risking disclosing too much, the one thing which is guaranteed to make me laugh is flatulence. Ideally someone else's. I can very quickly be reduced to that bone-shaking, tummy-hurting, tear-making, silent laughter in response to someone else's toot. All the better if it takes them by surprise too. I am chuckling to myself as I write this. There you have it. I am not sure if I should be ashamed that my sense of humour has not progressed much beyond that of a six year old.

But what about outside work? What makes you happy in your non-work life?

If you want to know about my non-work life then the things that make me most happy are my family, my cat, gardening, and being outdoors.

I moved back to the Chichester area in 2021 so I could spend more time with my family (who are all based in West Sussex). I wanted to play a more active role in the lives of my young niece and nephews. I love to spend time with them and really value seeing the world anew through their eyes. They call me their 'Weird Auntie Karen' and I think that, out of all my titles, that is my favourite.

I accidentally became a cat lover when I took in my dad's cats after he died. Within a couple of months, they had stolen my heart and had the house running in the way that best suited them. My transformation was as much a surprise to me as it was to my family. To mark them getting under my skin, I went and got myself a tattoo (or 'cattoo' as I call it!).

I know very little about gardening, but I love to potter about. The garden I took on when I bought my house was fairly small. Just grass (with dog pee patches). I took all the grass out, made some paths (even hiring a 'thumpy-thumpy' machine to pack down the paths I was making) and began to add plants and, most recently, a small pond. Nearly four years since beginning the transformation, it is taking shape and is full of birds, bees, and insects. There is nothing better than coming home and sitting in the garden with a cup of tea and letting the day's stresses melt away. Being outdoors always recharges me – even on wet and windy days.

So now you know a bit about what makes me tick. But although some of that information might be of interest, it does not really explain why I feel I can write a book about how to live well with persistent pain does it?

WHY SHOULD WE LISTEN TO WHAT SHE HAS TO SAY? WHAT DOES SHE KNOW ABOUT PERSISTENT PAIN?

In my opinion, it is the experiences we have after qualifying that make us most qualified. It is like learning to drive. It is not really until you have passed the test and been driving for some time that you really learn about driving and driving well. So I will start by mentioning my qualifications and then I will move on to sharing my experiences so you can make a judgement about whether you want to read on through this book.

What are your qualifications?

I have academic, practitioner, and teaching qualifications. I have also worked closely with the organisation that is my professional body, and I have been recognised by them for my work.

Academic

I have a degree in psychology. This means I can have the letters BSc (Hons) after my name. I have also been awarded a doctorate. This is the highest educational qualification you can study for. It is also known as a PhD. A PhD is a really big piece of research that you plan, do, and write up. Once you have written up the research, it is assessed by other experts in your field. They interview you over a number of hours to check you really did the work and that you know what you are talking about. They then decide whether or not you have passed. When you complete your doctorate, you can use the letters 'PhD' after your name.

Practitioner

I am a qualified health psychologist. I am registered with the Health and Care Professions Council (HCPC). The HCPC is the professional body that makes sure people who work as psychologists are qualified to do so. They also make sure that we keep our skills up to date and check that we are safe to practise.

Professional body

I have been actively involved with my professional body, the British Psychological Society (BPS). I started out as a member of the BPS Division of Health Psychology Committee. I became the committee's honorary secretary for a few years. I co-hosted a huge joint conference with our European sister society: the European Health Psychology Society (EHPS). And then, in 2014, I was elected chair of the BPS Division of Health Psychology. I spent a year as chair elect, two years as chair, and one year as 'past chair'.

I am a chartered psychologist. The 'chartered' status means I have been deemed to have reached the highest standard of psychological knowledge and expertise. I can put the letters 'CPsychol' after my name. I am an also an elected fellow of the BPS. A fellowship recognises the significant contribution made to the advancement or communication of psychological knowledge or practice by research, teaching, publications, or public service, or by organising and developing the work of others. This is the highest designation the society can bestow, showing a person's significant contribution and understanding of the discipline. With this, I can add more letters after my name as, as a fellow, a person is entitled to use 'FBPsS'.

Teaching

I am a senior fellow of the Higher Education Academy (HEA). Being recognised as a fellow means I have demonstrated a personal commitment to professionalism in learning and teaching in higher education. This also means I can put the letters 'SFHEA' after my name.

So I have a lot of letters after my name:

Dr Karen Rodham, BSc (Hons), PhD, CPsychol, FBPsS, SFHEA

BUT WHAT HAVE YOU DONE WITH THESE QUALIFICATIONS?

Gaining qualifications is all well and good, but the important thing is what you do with them. What experiences have you gained since qualifying? Have you used your qualifications for good? I will let you decide as I share some of my post-qualification experiences.

Teaching

Most of my career has been spent training the next generation of psychologists. I have been teaching in universities since 1995. I started out working mostly with undergraduate students and shifted to working with those completing their postgraduate training and now spend a lot of time training the next generation of health psychologists.

Researching

If I were to try to sum up my research, I would say that I have spent my life trying to understand how we can better help people to live well when they also live with long-term physical health conditions. I want to hear their stories in their own words. I want to understand how *they* want to be helped, not how I think they could or should be helped.

Practice

From 2006 to 2013 I worked part time in the NHS (UK National Health Service) in a pain-management service at (what used to be called) The Royal National Hospital for Rheumatic Diseases in Bath, United Kingdom. I worked part time as a health psychologist in the complex regional pain syndrome (CRPS) service. I designed a psychology service that would complement the approaches of the other members of the multidisciplinary team and spent the next six years dividing my time between the university and hospital. It was a privilege working with such an amazing team of lovely human beings. I learned so much from all the people who were living with CRPS.

Writing

I have written journal articles and books on a range of topics. In terms of persistent pain, the work I have done on CRPS was used in the National CRPS Guidelines. I wrote a leaflet for the charity Pain Concern about coping with CRPS. When I finished working at the hospital, I wrote a book sharing all I had learned from the people living with CRPS (Rodham, 2015). I also wrote a book about pain self-management (Rodham, 2020).

SO WHAT DO YOU THINK? NOW YOU KNOW ME A LITTLE BETTER, DO YOU TRUST ME ENOUGH TO READ ON?

I hope that this start to my book helps you feel you know me a little better. You now know about my qualifications and experience, so I hope that you can see I am qualified on paper *and* through experience to talk about the things I want to discuss in this book. I am an academic and a practitioner. I do not want to keep my learning all to myself – I want to find ways to share it with others. I hope this book does exactly that.

And I hope you will choose to read on.

ACKNOWLEDGEMENTS

To the people living with pain with whom I have sat alongside, as together we looked for ways to live life well in spite of the pain: I owe you a huge debt. You have taught me so much.

To the research and practice worlds: Thank you for your generosity in sharing your wisdom and for continuing to do so even as our practice and academic worlds become metricised and ever more demanding.

To Routledge, Taylor & Francis Group, and the British Psychological Society: Thank you for trusting and encouraging me to write this book.

To Florence and Sue who have edited this book and, in so doing, have taught me much about how to improve my writing.

To the anonymous reviewers: Thank you. Your constructive feedback strengthened my proposal.

To my friends: Thank you for the wisdom, the laughter, and above all the smut and nonsense.

To my neighbours Phillip and Stephen: Thank you for the delicious meals, fine wine, lovely company, and always interesting conversations. I am blessed to have you as next door neighbours.

And, above all, to my family, without whom life is meaningless: Thank you for being there, for boosting my confidence, yet keeping my feet firmly on the ground, and for bringing me cups of tea when I spent my weekends in the library writing. Being 'Weird Auntie Karen' is my favourite ever role.

FURTHER RESOURCES

PROFESSIONAL BODIES

British Psychological Society. https://www.bps.org.uk/chartered-membership-cpsychol [accessed 11 May 2025].

Division of Health Psychology. https://www.bps.org.uk/member-networks/division-health-psychology [accessed 10 January 2026].

European Health Psychology Society. https://ehps.net/ [accessed 10 January 2026].

Health and Care Professions Council. https://www.hcpc-uk.org/ [accessed 11 May 2025].

Higher Education Academy. https://www.advance-he.ac.uk/fellowship [accessed 11 May 2025].

Complex Regional Pain Syndrome guidelines. https://www.rcp.ac.uk/improving-care/resources/complex-regional-pain-syndrome-in-adults-2nd-edition/ [accessed 10 January 2026].

Complex Regional Pain Syndrome leaflet. https://painconcern.org.uk/complex-regional-pain-syndrome-leaflet/ [accessed 10 January 2026].

REFERENCES

Rodham, K. (2015). *Learning to cope with CRPS: Putting life first and pain second*. Singing Dragon.

Rodham, K. (2020). *Self-management for persistent pain: The blame, shame and inflame game?* Palgrave Macmillan.

1

WHAT IS PERSISTENT PAIN?

WHY IS IT IMPORTANT THAT WE LEARN ABOUT IT?

INTRODUCTION

Pain, for many people, is something fleeting. This kind of pain lasts as long as it takes to fix the injury. This kind of pain is called 'acute' pain. In my well-thumbed *Concise Oxford Dictionary* (1989), the word 'acute' is defined as 'coming sharply to a crisis'. Acute pain is a normal part of our everyday life and, as noted by Eccleston and colleagues (2023, p. 1), can include anything from a 'momentary muscular cramp to post-operative pain'. Think about how often you to stub your toe, have a headache, experience muscle cramp, bruise yourself because you bumped into the corner of the table (again!). In other words, acute pain is a really common human experience. However, for increasing numbers of people, pain is not something acute that reaches a crisis and subsides, it stays (persists) for longer than would be expected. The British Pain Society suggest that, in the United Kingdom, almost half of us will experience chronic pain. Returning to my trusty dictionary, the word 'chronic' is defined as 'lingering, lasting, bad, intense, severe'. And it is this chronic, persistent type of pain that this book focuses upon.

In this chapter I will explain how persistent pain is defined and give an overview of how pain is caused. I will also explain how researchers

DOI: 10.4324/9781003649854-1

and clinicians have approached the challenge of measuring pain, and I will share some figures to give you an insight into how common persistent pain is. My intention is to provide you with some context that will help you see that persistent pain is an extremely important issue. Not just for those who live with persistent pain, but for their loved ones, their colleagues, and the health professionals who work with them to help them cope with their persistent pain.

HOW IS PAIN DEFINED?

On one level it seems very straightforward. We know when we are in pain. We can say that our pain hurts, and we may be able to point to where we are experiencing the pain in our body. But we cannot touch pain itself. Raja and colleagues (2020) quote Sir Thomas Lewis as having written: 'Reflection tells me that I am so far from being able to define pain that the attempt could serve no useful purpose.' This captures the difficulty of trying to define something we experience yet is not visible and so is not measurable objectively. Pincus and Sheikh (2014, p. 2) describe the experience of pain as being 'like a visit from a ghost, pain comes and goes in its own unpredictable manner invisible and undetectable by others, including the best modern medical technology'. In other words, pain is an experience. It is our experience, and this makes it something that is unique to us. Pain is therefore something that is both complicated and invisible, and so it is a really difficult thing to define. The difficulty of capturing the essence of pain in a simple definition is clear when you look at the (revised) definition of pain that was published in 2020 by the International Association for the Study of Pain (IASP, 2020). Pain is described in one sentence, but it also needs six extra notes to further explain this sentence. The definition (which can be found on the IASP website and in a paper by Raja et al., 2020) states that pain is an 'unpleasant sensory and emotional experience associated with, or resembling that associated with, actual or potential tissue damage'. This means that pain is 'not nice' – and it is not just physical, but also emotionally distressing. The definition also makes it clear that we can experience pain when our bodies are damaged *and* when we think that they might be damaged. Already this one sentence is sharing some complex explanations. But, as I have mentioned, the definition also has six extra notes to give context to the definition. I have summarised them below:

- Pain is something that is unique to each of us. Many different things can influence how we experience pain. These include our biology, our psychology, and our social situations.
- Our body has pain detective systems (called nociceptors) that keep a watch out for things that could damage our body. When our nociceptors identify a threat, they send a signal to our brain. It is our brain that decodes the signal and decides whether the threat is, or could be, painful.
- Our life experiences and culture teach us how to respond to pain. These experiences are used by our brain when it is working out how to respond to the nociceptor signals.
- If someone says they are in pain, they should be both believed and respected.
- Although pain can be useful because it moves us away from harm, pain can impact negatively on our wellbeing.
- There are a lot of different ways to express pain. If a human or animal cannot describe their pain, we should not assume that they are not in pain.

IF PAIN IS DIFFICULT TO DEFINE, HOW IS PERSISTENT OR CHRONIC PAIN DEFINED?

Given how complicated it seems to be to define pain, is it any easier to define persistent or chronic pain? In a recent update to the International Classification of Diseases (ICD), chronic pain was split into two types: 'chronic primary' or 'chronic secondary' pain (Treede et al., 2019). Chronic primary pain is described as pain that has lasted for longer than three months and brings with it emotional distress, and/or the pain interferes with daily and social life, and the pain cannot be explained by another chronic condition. In other words, chronic primary pain is considered to be a disease. Examples that fit this definition include complex regional pain syndrome and fibromyalgia. In contrast, chronic secondary pain is defined as pain that is a symptom of another disease. Examples include pain related to cancer, surgery, and injury.

Researchers have also been trying to identify differences in the pain experience. For example, Eccleston and colleagues (2023) published a paper suggesting that acute and chronic pain could each be high or low in impact, and they explored how people might move between these states. Eccleston and colleagues' (2023) chronic pain high-impact category is, to my mind, very similar in definition to that of the ICD's chronic primary pain category. Both these approaches to defining long-lasting pain mention that for the pain to be defined as persistent (rather than acute), it needs to last longer than three months. However, three months is an arbitrary cut-off that has different impacts at different life stages. Eccleston and colleagues (2023) use the example of newborn babies who, as part of normal practice, have multiple tiny blood samples taken. These are called needlesticks. Each needlestick pain might be acute but, in terms of life context, that acute pain will have been present for most of the child's life. For a baby, three months is not a short duration. In other words, acute pain can also have a major impact on an individual. So defining persistent pain is complex. For the purposes of this book, when I use the phrase 'persistent pain', I will be referring to the WHO (2021) 'chronic primary pain' definition. In other words:

> Chronic (or persistent) pain is pain that has lasted for longer than three months which is accompanied by significant emotional distress and/or the pain interferes with daily and social life and the pain cannot be explained by another chronic condition.

Having shared some definitions of pain, we move our attention to the theories that have tried to offer an explanation for our pain experience.

WHAT DO THE THEORIES SAY ABOUT HOW WE FEEL PAIN?

Our understanding of the experience of pain continues to evolve. Originally pain was thought to come from pain receivers that sent a pain message to the brain through the spinal cord (Trout, 2004). Since then, the understanding we have of pain has become more nuanced as multiple influences on our experience of pain have been recognised. Indeed, the Gate-Control Theory, developed by Melzack and Wall (1965) was the first to link the psychological with the physiological processes in pain perception. In other words, this model suggested that pain was an experience or a perception that could only be experienced through an interaction between the mind (psychology) and the body (physiology). Pincus and Sheikh (2014) explain that the 'gate' (thought to be in the spinal cord) was the connection between the mind and the body. Psychological factors were thought to move down towards the gate and physiological signals to move up towards the gate. It was the intensity of the pain experience that opened the gate and sent the message to the brain to be decoded. In other words, the brain and body worked together. An example of how the brain and body work together might help here. McAllister (2015) suggests we think about what happens when we are children and we fall and graze our knees. Assuming the knee scrape is minor, if a trusted adult shows the child that they can see that they have hurt themselves (perhaps by giving the child a plaster), and then reassures them that they are all better now, before encouraging them to go back to their game, the child will learn that minor bumps are normal and nothing to worry about. Such a supportive interaction, which recognises the child's fear, does not downplay their pain experience yet reassures them that they will be fine. The message this conveys is that, although it hurts, it will not stop them from carrying on with their day. This positive and reassuring interaction changes the way the child's brain will respond to future bumps and scrapes.

In a TEDx talk,[1] Lorimer Moseley (2011) gives a different example of how our body and brain are connected when working out how to respond to a potentially painful experience. He is a very good 'teller of stories'. He talks of walking in the Australian countryside, when he experiences a painful sensation. He notices it and dismisses it as just a scratch from a twig. He carries on walking, takes a swim in the river and, after his swim, he passes out. It turns out he had been bitten by a brown snake. These snakes are very poisonous and being bitten is very serious. He is treated and gets well. Some time later, he is again walking in the Australian countryside. Again, he experiences a painful sensation. This time, the pain is intense and stops him in his tracks. He is convinced he has been bitten again. However, it turns out that the pain this time *was* started by a scratch from a twig. The take-home message is that our brain interprets and influences how we respond to pain signals.

HOW COMMON IS PERSISTENT PAIN?

Persistent pain is said to affect between a third and a half of the world's population and is the most common reason for accessing health care services (Kang et al., 2023). Liang (2024) notes that in 2019 in the United States, over 50 million adults experienced persistent pain and 24 million people endured work and life limitations because of persistent pain. In Spain, one in four Spanish people are affected by persistent pain (Dueñas et al., 2025). In Italy, one in five of the adult population experiences persistent pain (Violini et al., 2025). The estimated prevalence of persistent pain in the United States is also one in five (Rometsch et al., 2025). Shetty and colleagues (2024) note that 22 per cent of all primary care consultations in Finland are linked to persistent pain. The Faculty of Pain Medicine in the United Kingdom estimates that 43 per cent of adults live with a degree of persistent pain and suggests that persistent pain may affect up to 30 per cent of young adults of working age (18–39-year-olds). Indeed, in an effort to understand more about those living with persistent pain, Shetty and colleagues (2024) looked at the primary care records of over 300,000 people living in South London. They found that compared to other long-term conditions, people with chronic pain saw their general practitioners (GPs) more often. They also noted that there were differences in terms of gender (13.6 per cent males vs 24 per cent females) and ethnicity (17.5 per cent White and 27.2 per cent Black patients). Their study highlights the importance of looking beyond the overall headline number of people impacted. If we do this, we can better understand whether some groups of people might be more affected by chronic pain. For example, if we look at age, gender, social deprivation, and ethnicity (Anderson et al., 2020; Grol-Prokopeczyk, 2017; Versus Arthritis, 2021), we identify groups who are more likely to experience persistent pain.

Age

Dueñas and colleagues (2025) report that the prevalence of persistent pain in Spain was highest in the group aged between 57 and 75 years. Similarly, in their review of European adult populations, Rometsch and colleagues (2025) report that persistent pain was more prevalent in the older age groups (45–64 and over 65 years). The UK Faculty of Pain Medicine states that the prevalence of persistent pain in older age groups is higher than the national average of 43 per cent, with up to 62 per cent of those aged 75 years and older reporting persistent pain.

Gender

Females are more likely to report or experience persistent pain than males (Biring et al., 2025; Mills et al., 2019; Rice et al., 2024), more likely to experience severe, disabling pain than males of a similar age (Versus Arthritis, 2021), and are more likely to experience chronic pain conditions that are not straightforward to diagnose or treat (e.g., fibromyalgia). Rice and colleagues (2024) argue that this means that women's pain is more often minimised and disbelieved (e.g., Quintner, 2020). Furthermore, Keogh (2025) notes that women experience more pain across a range of conditions over their lifespan. There are also gender differences in terms of how we tell health professionals about our pain. For example, one study found that men were less likely to report pain if they were with a male friend (Edwards et al., 2017), and another study showed that patients report pain in different ways when they speak to male or female health care professionals (Vigil & Alcock, 2014).

Social Deprivation

It is well known that low socioeconomic status (SES) is a risk factor for health problems (Dirksen et al., 2022; Zaneva et al., 2024). Typically, SES is measured by a person's education, income, job, social class, and assets. For example, in America, Cutler and colleagues (2020) reported a clear socioeconomic gradient in knee pain experience by age and education. They found that those aged 60–64 years with less education were more likely to report pain that impacted on their activities of daily living. In Austria, Dorner and colleagues (2010) showed that those people who lived in less wealthy areas reported a higher prevalence of pain compared to those who lived in more wealthy areas. Those who were unemployed had the highest prevalence of pain, the highest level of feeling strongly disabled through pain, and the highest intensity of pain. Similarly, a team from Spain and Tehran conducted a review of published work and concluded that socioeconomic status was an important predictor of both the occurrence and severity of persistent pain. They also suggest that the prevalence of persistent pain is twice as high in low- and middle-income countries compared to high-income countries (Prego-Dominguez et al., 2021).

Ethnicity

A disparity in the health status of African Americans over their lifespan has been highlighted by Maly and Vallerand (2018). They note that this population had a higher prevalence of chronic pain, worse chronic pain outcomes, and poorer treatment of chronic pain. They also showed that African Americans living in urban poverty lacked safe access to physical activity, had decreased social support because of neighbourhood characteristics, and faced increased exposure to neighbourhood violence; all of which had a cumulative influence on their experience of chronic pain. For example, for those living in poverty, low socioeconomic status haunts each financial decision. Many were unable to consistently afford prescribed medicine or travel costs for visits to health care providers to manage their pain. Similarly, Walker-Taylor and colleagues (2018) note that older African Americans report more unresolved pain than other racial/ethnic groups and less control over their pain.

There is also evidence to show that we are not collecting the right information to allow us to judge whether we are meeting the needs of people from minority ethnic groups. Leach and colleagues (2024) reviewed the literature and noted that some studies only recorded 'White British' (and made no mention of other ethnicities), and no studies had specifically assessed ethnic disparities within chronic pain services. Until these data are collected, it will be not be possible to identify inequality in accessing services.

Leach and colleagues (2024) also highlighted two contradictory findings in their review. First, that there was evidence to show that self-reported pain was more common among minority ethnic groups in the United Kingdom (e.g., Choudhury et al., 2013). Second, that use of outpatient chronic pain services is significantly lower among minority ethnic groups compared to White British. If these two figures are true, and chronic pain services were accessible to everyone, then we would expect a larger proportion of minority ethnic groups to access chronic pain services (see Clementi, 2020). The limited representation of ethnicity identified by Leach and colleagues (2024, p. 3504) is not uncommon despite there being 'general agreement that ethnicity data collection is essential to better understand and reduce disparities in healthcare, given it has been suggested that structural racism is a potential public health risk within the UK'. Of course, none of us belong to just one group, so we also need to be mindful of intersectionality, in other words, the impact of belonging to multiple groups. For example, Bonathan and colleagues (2013, p. 161) conclude:

> The consequences of feeling socially inferior, living in a less socially cohesive neighbourhood with a more imminent sense of threat, combined with poorer education and therefore poorer job opportunities are likely to interact with the psychological factors known to increase the risk of chronic pain.

Likewise, Maly and Vallerand (2018) note that we need to better assess the risk factors that make chronic pain both more likely and more severe, including biological, environmental, health care system, and cultural factors. For example, older and middle-aged African American women are at a particularly high risk of experiencing pain and pain-related disability because of the intersection of their sex, age, race, and high rates of chronic conditions such as osteoarthritis (Walker-Taylor et al., 2018). This ties in with the work of Michael Marmot (2015) who uses the term 'status syndrome' to highlight how inequality in power, money, and resources (at the individual, local, national, and global level) give rise to inequalities in daily life that in turn give rise to inequalities in health.

SO WHY IS IT IMPORTANT TO LEARN ABOUT PERSISTENT PAIN?

This chapter has explained what persistent pain is and how common it is. The UK Faculty of Pain Medicine suggests that there is likely to be a growth in the numbers of new cases of chronic pain of 32 per cent by the year 2040. Persistent pain is the top reason to seek care and the top cause of disability. It affects millions of people worldwide and is leading to personal and societal burdens (see Fricton et al., 2025). In other words, if we do not experience it ourselves, someone we know will. We should all take an interest in this and learn about it so we can better help ourselves, our loved ones, and our colleagues when living with persistent pain.

WHAT ARE THE COMMON QUESTIONS PEOPLE ASK ABOUT PERSISTENT PAIN?

This chapter concludes with a set of common questions people ask when thinking about persistent pain, each of which will be addressed in a separate chapter.

- What is it like to live with persistent pain?
- Why is it so hard to explain persistent pain to someone else?
- Why is it so hard to manage your own pain?
- Is it true that laughter and swearing can help with pain?
- What has psychology got to do with persistent pain?
- So what can we all do to help those who live with persistent pain, live well in spite of their persistent pain?

FURTHER RESOURCES

Professional bodies

The British Pain Society. https://www.britishpainsociety.org/ [accessed 10 January 2026].

European Pain Federation (EFIC). https://europeanpainfederation.eu/ [accessed 10 January 2026].

International Association for the Study of Pain. https://www.iasp-pain.org/about/ [accessed 10 January 2026].

World Health Organization (WHO), International Classification of Diseases (ICD). https://icd.who.int/en/ [accessed 10 January 2026].

Useful talks

Prof. Tamar Pincus video explaining pain: This is an excellent video explaining what it is like to live with persistent pain. Patients I used to work with, found this video useful. https://youtu.be/ZUXPqphwp2U?feature=shared [accessed 10 January 2026].

Lorimer Mosely Ted talk: The example I refer to in the chapter is described in the first five minutes of the talk. https://www.youtube.com/watch?v=gwd-wLdIHjs [accessed 10 January 2026].

NOTE

1 TED (Technology, Education, and Design) is a non-profit organisation that brings together expert thinkers and doers to share new ideas. TEDx talks (the 'x' stands for independently organised) are local events that bring people together to share new ideas in the style of global TED talks. [See https://conferences.ted.com/.]

REFERENCES

Anderson, S.R., Gianola, M., Perry, J.M., and Losin, E.A. (2020). Clinician-patient racial/ethnic concordance influences racial/ethnic minority pain: Evidence from simulated clinical interactions. *Pain Medicine*, 21(11), 3109–3125.

Biring, S., Burton, A.E., Dunwoody, L., and Kevern, P. (2025). Women's experiences of living with chronic pain: A qualitative meta-synthesis. *British Journal of Health Psychology*, 30, e70023. https://doi.org/10.1111/bjhp.70023.

Bonathan, C., Hearn, L., and C de C Williams, A. (2013). Socioeconomic status and the course and consequences of pain. *Pain Management*, 3(3), 159–162.

Choudhury, Y., Bremner, S.A., Ali, A., et al. (2013). Prevalence and impact of chronic widespread pain in the Bangladeshi and White populations of Tower Hamlets East London. *Clinical Rheumatology*, 32, 1375–1382.

Clementi, R. (2020). Structural racism remains a primary public health risk amidst COVID and beyond in the United Kingdom. *Journal of Public Health*, 42(3). https://doi.org/10.1093/pubmed/fdaa102.

Concise Oxford Dictionary (1989). *The Concise Oxford Dictionary of Current English* (7th edition). Oxford University Press.

Cutler, D.M., Meara, E., and Stewart, S. (2020). Socioeconomic status and the experience of pain: An example from knees. *NBER Working Paper Series*, Working Paper 27974. http://www.nber.org/papers/w27974.

Dirksen, J., Pinilla-Ronancio, M., Wehrmeister, F.C., et al. (2022). Exploring the potential for a new measure of socioeconomic deprivation status to monitor health inequality. *International Journal for Equity in Health*, https://.doi.org/10.1186/s12939-022-01661-0.

Dorner, T.E., Muckenhuber, J., Stronegger, W.J., et al. (2010). The impact of socio-economic status on pain and the perception of disability due to pain. *European Journal of Pain*, 15, 103–109.

Dueñas, M., De Sola, H., Salazar, A., et al. (2025). Prevalence and epidemiological characteristics of chronic pain in the Spanish population. Results from the pain barometer. *European Journal of Pain*, 29, e4705. https://doi.org/10.1002/ejp.4705.

Eccleston, C., Begley, E., Birkinshaw, H., et al. (2023). The establishment, maintenance, and adaptation of high- and low-impact chronic pain: A framework for biopsychosocial pain research. *Pain*. http://dx.doi.org/10.1097/j.pain.0000000000002951.

Edwards, R., Eccleston, C., and Keogh, E. (2017). Observer influences on pain: An experimental series examining same-sex and opposite-sex friends, strangers, and romantic partners. *Pain*, 158(5), 846–855.

Faculty of Pain Medicine website: https://fpm.ac.uk/ [accessed 28 January 2026].

Fricton, J., Lawson, K., Gerwin, R., and Shueb, S. (2025). Preventing chronic pain: Solutions to a public health crisis. *Igmin Research*, 3(1), 038–051.

Grol-Prokopeczyk, H. (2017). Sociodemographic disparities in chronic pain, based on 12-year longitudinal data. *Pain*, 158(2), 313–322.

International Association for the Study of Pain (IASP) (2020). https://www.iasp-pain.org/about/ [accessed 10 January 2026].

Kang, Y., Trewern, L. Jackman, J., et al. (2023). Chronic pain: Definitions and diagnosis. *BMJ*, 381, e076036. http://dx.doi.org/10.1136/bmj-2023-076036.

Keogh, E. (2025). Sex, gender and pain: Evidence and knowledge gaps. *Current Opinion in Psychology*, 63, 102006. https://doi.org/10.1016/j.copsyc.2025.102006.

Leach, E., Ndosi, M., and Jones, G.T. (2024). Access to chronic pain services for adults from minority ethnic groups in the United Kingdom (UK): A scoping review. *Journal of Racial and Ethnic Health Disparities*, 11, 3498–3508.

Liang, Y. (2024). Life course socioeconomic status, chronic pain, and the mediating role of allostatic load: Findings from the midlife in the United States. *Frontiers in Public Health*, 12, 1365105.

Maly, A. and Vallerand, A.H. (2018). Neighborhood, socioeconomic, and racial influence on chronic pain. *Pain Management Nursing*, 19(1), 14–22.

Marmot, M. (2015). *Status syndrome: How your social standing directly affects your health and life expectancy*. Bloomsbury Publishing (9781408872680).

McAllister, M. (2015). What is the neuromatrix of pain? *What is Chronic Pain?* https://www.instituteforchronicpain.org/understanding-chronic-pain/what-is-chronic-pain/neuromatrix-of-pain [2023; accessed 10 January 2026].

Melzack, R. and Wall, P.D. (1965). Pain mechanisms: A new theory. *Science*, 150(3699), 971–979.

Mills, S.E.E., Nicolson, K.P. and Smith, B.H. (2019). Chronic pain: a review of its epidemiology and associated factors in population-based studies. *British Journal of Anaesthesia*, 123(2), e273–e283.

Moseley, L. (2011): https://www.youtube.com/watch?v=gwd-wLdIHjs [accessed 10 January 2026].

Pincus, D. and Sheikh, A.A. (2014). *Imagery for pain relief: A scientifically grounded guidebook for clinicians*. Routledge.

Prego-Dominguez, J.P., Khazaeipour, Z., Mallah, N., and Takkouche, B. (2021). Socioeconomic status and occurrence of chronic pain: a meta-analysis. *Rheumatology*, 60, 1091–1105.

Quintner, J. (2020). Why are women with fibromyalgia so stigmatized? *Pain Medicine*, 21, 882–888.

Raja, S.N., Carr, D.B., Cohen, M., et al. (2020). The revised IASP definition of pain: Concepts, challenges and compromises. *Pain*, 161(9), 1978–1982.

Rice, K., Connoy, L., and Webster, F. (2024). Gendered worlds of pain: Women, marginalization and chronic pain. *The Journal of Pain*, 11, 104626

Rometsch, C., Martin, A., Junne, F., and Cosci, F. (2025). Chronic pain in European adult populations: A systematic review of prevalence and associated clinical features. *Pain*, 166, 719–731.

Shetty, S., Scuffell, J., Aitken, D., and Ashworth, M. (2024). Chronic pain:prevalence, demographic inequalities and healthcare utilisation: a primary care database analysis. *British Journal of General Practice*, https://doi.org/10.3399/BJGPO.2024.0147.

The British Pain Society website: https://www.britishpainsociety.org/ [accessed 28 January 2026].

Treede, R.D., Rief, W., Barke, A. et al. (2019). Chronic pain as a symptom or a disease: the IASP classification of chronic pain for the International Classification of Diseases (ICD-11). *Pain*, 160, 19–27.

Trout, K.K. (2004). The neuromatrix theory of pain: Implications for selected non-pharmacological methods of pain relief for labor. *Journal of Midwifery and Women's Health*, 49(6), 482–488.

Versus Arthritis (2021). *Chronic pain in England: Unseen, unequal, unfair*. Versus Arthritis.

Vigil, J.M. and Alcock, J. (2014). Tough guys or sensitive guys? Disentangling the role of examiner sex on patient pain reports. *Pain Research Management*, 19(1), e9–e12.

Violini, A., Consoletti, L., and Finco, G. (2025). Chronic pain in Italy: Turning numbers into actionable solutions. *Pain Research and Management*, https://doi.org/10.1155/prm/3401242.

Walker-Taylor, J.L., Campbell, C.M., Thorpe, R.J., et al. (2018). Pain, racial discrimination, and depressive symptoms among African American women. *Pain Management Nursing*, 19(1), 79–87.

World Health Organization (WHO) (2021). International Classification of Diseases (ICD) resource: https://icd.who.int/en/ [accessed 10 January 2020].

Zaneva, M., Dumbalska, T., Reeves, A., and Bowes, L. (2024). What do we mean when we talk about socioeconomic status? Implications for measurement, mechanisms, and interventions from a critical review on adolescent mental health. *General Psychiatry*, 37: e101455.

2

WHAT IS IT LIKE TO LIVE WITH PERSISTENT PAIN?

INTRODUCTION

Just like sight, sound, taste, touch, and smell, pain is also a sense (Drissi et al., 2020). We have special receptors in our body that help us to recognise (or sense) actual and potential damage to our body. These receptors play a key role in our experience of pain. However, there are some people who do not experience pain. They have what is called congenital insensitivity to pain (CIP). This is a rare condition. Schon and colleagues (2020) estimate that since there are fewer than 30 cases in the United Kingdom the chances of having CIP is one in a million.

Yippee! you might think. A life without pain. How marvellous. But if you stop for a moment and think about it, life would be quite tricky. After all, pain lets us know when we need to get out of dangerous situations (Itmaiza et al., 2025). Think about all the things in your kitchen that could do you harm if your pain system was not working. For example, if you were to absent-mindedly pick up a tray of roast potatoes that had just come out of the oven, your pain response system would step up and make you drop the tray very quickly. Quite likely it would stop you from even picking up the tray. As soon as your fingers touched the hot surface, your arm would jerk back. Someone with CIP would not feel the pain and would carry the

DOI: 10.4324/9781003649854-2

tray across the kitchen. Sounds all right so far – but, although they are not experiencing pain, their body is being damaged by the very hot tray. They will end up with a severe burn. Indeed, Corkhill (2021, p. 126) sums up the protective nature of pain: "Pain evolved to stop us keeping our hand in a hot fire and ensures we don't put it back a second time. It ensures we don't walk on a broken leg." So, as you can probably imagine, it is not surprising that people who have CIP repeatedly injure themselves. This was explored in 2017, when the BBC wrote an article called: 'The curse of the people who never feel pain'. In the article they share the experiences of 21-year-old Stefan who lives with CIP. He was quoted as saying:

> People assume that feeling no pain is this incredible thing and it almost makes you superhuman. For people with CIP it's the exact opposite. We would love to know what pain means and what it feels like to be in pain. Without it, your life is full of challenges.

Although this chapter is focused on what it is like to live with persistent pain, learning more about the experiences of those who are unable to feel pain could be really useful. Teams of researchers are trying to understand more about CIP because, if we can better understand what it is that turns off the ability to feel pain when a person has CIP, maybe new painkillers could be developed that would help those who are living with persistent pain.

So, unless you are one of those rare people who have no capacity to feel pain, you will know that pain brings challenges. Many of us will have experienced a stubbed toe, a broken bone, a toothache, a blister, a headache. These episodes of acute (short-lived) pain are unpleasant. Perhaps they lay us very low while they last, but they are temporary. We experience pain, but we know it will soon pass, the broken bone will mend, we might not be able to resist picking the blister but, even so, the skin will heal. Maybe we need to take a bit of time off work, maybe we just need to lie down in a darkened room till the headache passes. If we are lucky, we will receive sympathetic comments or perhaps even be sent get well soon cards from friends and family.

And then, when the pain has passed, we pick up more or less where we left off and move forward with our lives. But those people who experience persistent pain have a very different experience.

CHALLENGE 1: THE BEGINNING

Maybe it starts with an injury that just does not get better. Maybe it is something that you notice, but assume will go away. Then you realise a few weeks have passed, and the pain is still there. Not enough to trouble you too much, but enough to make things a bit more difficult than usual. Each person experiences things differently, but there are two things that people who live with persistent pain have in common (van Hout et al., 2023, p. 2). The first is that persistent pain comes to be "experienced as something which will never cease". The other is that persistent pain is both 'never changing' and 'ever changing'. In other words, although the pain is always there, the way in which the pain is experienced changes. This is explained by a participant in a study by Clarke and colleagues (2012, p. 4):

> Well, the average day is bad [laughs] the pain doesn't go away. But the time of day in which its worst, is between five o'clock and ten o'clock in the evening, even up to eleven o'clock. [...] There's no time when there's no pain. One is very light pain ... Two is a wee bit ... one, two, three, four, five, up to five o'clock is bearable [...]. Then it goes steadily up and also saps my energy. [Caucasian Female 1, aged 78, with joint pain.]

Trying to describe to someone else that the pain does not go away but that, at the same time, it also changes makes it difficult to explain. For example, another person who took part in Clarke and colleagues' study (2012, p. 4) said:

> It's there ever present, it's there right now and it's worse at some times than others. It's a very difficult thing to describe to you. I used to work in the dairy industry and we used refrigeration

> quite a lot, and if you listen to refrigeration going through pipes, that's exactly the same feeling as I have in my feet; it's a sort of a bubbling. [Caucasian Male 9, aged 68, with foot pain.]

If you can't find the words to explain your pain, how can you find help? But once you realise your pain is not going away, finding help is what you will need to do. You will begin your journey to diagnosis.

Challenge 2: The journey to diagnosis

The journey to diagnosis is often long and bumpy. It can take a long time to be referred to a pain expert. Anna, a participant in a study by Costa and colleagues (2023, p. 2752) spoke about her long wait in the Australian system:

> I was on the waiting list to see pain management for nearly two years. Finally got into two different places. One of them was going to be telehealth and I thought "will go with that one then I don't have to travel 200 kms to see somebody" and so I accepted that referral and then knocked back the other one. I did all the intake and then didn't hear anything. I'm thinking "what's going on?". So, following up on it, they've got defunded. Nobody bothered to let me know. So now I have to go back on the waitlist.

Anna's story is not unusual, and lengthy wait times are not unique to Australia. A study in Canada reported 22 per cent of adults in their survey saying they had waited for longer than a year for their pain clinic appointment (Liddy et al., 2024). Similarly, the King's Fund (2025) noted that waiting lists in the United Kingdom regularly miss the NHS (National Health Service) target of a maximum of 18 weeks. Obviously, waiting for an appointment is frustrating, but there are other impacts too. For example, waits of six months from the time of referral to treatment for chronic pain are known to have a negative impact on the quality of life and wellbeing of the person who is waiting. Indeed, in the light of their review of the existing evidence, Lynch and colleagues (2008) concluded that wait times for chronic pain treatment of six months or longer were medically unacceptable and that more work was needed to better understand at what point people began to get worse while waiting.

The search for a diagnosis, is not just about waiting for appointments. It is also about finding your way around a health system that, on one hand, acknowledges that pain is whatever the person experiencing the pain says it is (McCaffery, 1968) and, on the other, looks for objective measures of something that (as we have already noted) is both never changing and ever changing. As such, people experiencing persistent pain speak of the need to learn to speak up and become self-advocates. In a study exploring the experiences of young adults living with persistent pain, Karadag and colleagues (2025, p. 5) noticed that because participants did not feel that they were a priority, they had to learn take the initiative. One of their participants, Julie, said:

> [We need to] be proactive with doctors and stuff like that and chase them for their being slow and that is really difficult when you have chronic pain and everything's exhausting, but it's really important because a lot of the time, otherwise you get left to the side or left on some waiting list.

Living with persistent pain is difficult. Asking for help from the health profession, but feeling you are not being believed or properly listened to, makes things much worse. In their paper highlighting the experiences of those who were seeking a diagnosis, Kang and colleagues (2023) said that patients frequently felt as though they needed to defend their experience of severe pain. For example, a person I interviewed (Rodham, 2015, p. 30) said:

> They just do not believe you are in pain. They just can't see it. There's nothing. The pain is so disproportionate if you like, to the actual physical symptoms that they think "What are you

> playing at?" and sometimes you want to walk around with a plaque on saying "I'm in real pain here".

Similarly, Costa and colleagues (2023) interviewed 15 people in Australia who had had lower back pain for at least two years and were looking for help in understanding their pain. Once all the interviews were analysed it was clear that there were four key questions that were important to these participants: 'What will happen over time?', 'Can clinicians help me and are they willing to?', 'What are clinicians talking about?', and 'Am I being taken seriously?'. All four questions were linked by the overwhelming uncertainty they experienced as they tried to live with their persistent pain. For example, Jorge, aged 36 had been experiencing persistent pain for two years at the time of his interview. He was finding it difficult to cope with his GP's uncertainty about what was causing his pain:

> Frustrated again … I wasn't mentally or physically prepared to, or even emotionally prepared to start having a chronic condition. I was still hoping that it would be an acute condition. But as time passed, I sort of saw it progressing, the pain was still the same sometimes going up, going down, but not going away … the uncertainty of not knowing how this condition will resolve … And I'd say that, although I've been with pain for the last two years, I'm still poorly prepared to manage uncertainty.
>
> (Costa et al., 2023, p. 2752)

When you are looking for an explanation for your pain, you may well be sent for a range of tests. This is because the pain might be a symptom of something else and it is important to see if the cause can be identified. One participant in a study by Hadi and colleagues (2017) spoke about the multiple potential causes that were explored as part of their search for a diagnosis: 'I went to the doctors, it's nothing. Tennis elbow, then it was arthritis, then it wasn't arthritis, then it was because of a previous injury.' Indeed, having multiple tests can be an emotional roller-coaster. There may be the fear of what might be causing the pain, followed by the strangeness of being almost disappointed that a test for something serious comes up negative. After that there may be a feeling of guilt because of the disappointment experienced (even though the disappointment is about still having no explanation). Luke, aged 32 years at the time he was interviewed by Costa and colleagues (2023, p. 2752), had been living with lower back pain for 12 years. He spoke about the difficulty of coping with the uncertainty during the search for an explanation for his pain:

> The first confusion for me or uncertainty is the fact that I've had the same thing, the same type of pain come and go many, many times for many years, and then I was certain that something serious was going to come up on that test, but it didn't. So, it's like, okay, so I don't have anything, which is great. I don't have anything serious but this pain … this pain just can't be explained in a test. So that leaves me with this question in my head, because I know that it could come back at any time … and I still won't know, the actual reason why it happens, because the test came back with no issues at all.

Looking for an explanation for your pain but not finding one is very difficult to accept. Life can very quickly become focused on the next test. The more this becomes the focus, the more a person's life can shrink. While the search continues, some people begin to worry that if the pain cannot be explained by a test, then maybe their pain is all in their minds. I interviewed Crystal (Rodham, 2015, p. 73), who said: 'I really thought I was going mad and I thought I was making it up.' Others were told they might be imagining their pain. Hadi and colleagues (2017) interviewed a range of people in the United Kingdom, some of whom said that health professionals had told them that the pain was all in their minds:

> The second physiotherapist I saw basically told me that the pain was in my imagination. So I had one appointment with him. I'm

> in enough pain not to be able to tolerate people who are telling me it's not real, you know, because it is real. [Participant 10.]

The journey to diagnosis is therefore challenging. As well as managing your own uncertainty, while at the same time trying to find out what it is that is causing your pain, you also need to learn how to manage the responses of other people.

CHALLENGE 3: MANAGING OTHER PEOPLE'S RESPONSES DURING THE JOURNAL TO DIAGNOSIS

Living with persistent pain also involves managing other people's responses. If health professionals are suggesting the pain is all in the mind, it would not be surprising if friends, family and colleagues had similar thoughts. Indeed, Van Hout and colleagues (2023) have written about how people with persistent pain have friends, family, and health professionals who interpret their physical pain as being 'all in their head'. With persistent pain being invisible and difficult to describe, it is also difficult for other people to understand. This means that the person living with persistent pain is faced with managing their own responses to their situation *and* the responses of those around them – particularly health professionals and friends and family (e.g., De Ruddere et al., 2012; De Ruddere and Craig, 2016).

Health professionals

Upshur and colleagues (2010) recruited 72 adults living with chronic pain from primary care practices in Massachusetts and invited them to share their care experiences by taking part in group interviews. Many stories were shared describing experiences with health professionals whom participants felt did not 'fully respect, trust, support, and to believe the participants' reports of the severity and adverse effects of their pain'. Participants spoke of being labelled as hypochondriacs or of being accused of drug-seeking or even lying about their pain experiences. When the people to whom you turn for help do not support you, it is very difficult to continue to ask for help. Participants spoke about how the system made them feel like a burden. For example, a participant from Upshur and colleagues' (2020, p. 1793) study said:

> I show up before time then I have to sit in a room another half an hour while he is attending to 10 other patients at one time ... then he comes in and asked me 'how are you feeling, how is your pain? ... Okay. I'll fill the prescription' and in 5 minutes I am at the door ... I'm in there for 2 hours, he comes and gives me a prescription and kicks me out the door and says I'll see you in 3 months.

In the United Kingdom patients also report feeling that health professionals were not interested in their persistent pain. They also felt their health professionals lacked expertise in persistent pain. They felt that health professionals made an assumption that since chronic pain was not life threatening there was no need to identify the cause. Participant 9 (Hadi et al., 2017, p. 5) summed this up when they said: 'I don't know whether that's a cost thing, whether arthritis is not a sexy disease like cancer or other things that the NHS wants to throw money at.' In short, they felt that it would be a waste of time trying to explain their problem to health professionals, because it felt as though no one was interested in listening to them. This sounds like a lonely place to be.

Adding another layer to the negative experience was the feeling that there was no one who was keeping track of all the tests and appointments. Only the patient had an understanding of the bigger picture. The system was experienced as fragmented. They were sent to multiple specialists, none of whom seemed to communicate with one another. One participant in a study by Hadi and colleagues (2017, p. 4) was quoted as saying:

> I think you see everyone in isolation. So the physio will refer and they will write you a little letter and they will refer to a podiatrist. But then the podiatrist kind of sees the problem from

> such a different light that they're not really communicating with each other.

The lack of communication between specialists could have serious consequences, as shown in this extract from an interview with a participant (Hadi et al., 2017, p. 4) who had been prescribed medication for pain, apparently without regard to their other condition:

> The GP was worried about the high blood pressure, but didn't take time to look at the medication she'd actually put me on, whereas the pharmacist pointed it out to her. Potentially, according to the pharmacist, for three months, I was at high risk of having a stroke.

The lack of connection between and within services was seen as a huge challenge. This perspective was summed up by another participant who said:

> Within the NHS, every individual is great and they work really hard and they're really supportive, but they seem to be very caught in their little boxes and can't or aren't allowed to step outside them to maybe provide a more effective solution sometimes.
>
> (Hadi et al., 2017, p. 5)

Friends and family

LaForge (2025) interviewed 20 American people living with persistent pain. For many of them, family were key providers of support, but were also often experienced as judgemental. One participant in the study spoke of feeling supported by her husband and family, while at the same time, she felt she had failed her family. She said: 'I always fall short. … as a wife … as a daughter.' Others spoke about how the way in which they had grown up impacted on how they felt they should behave as an adult living with persistent pain: 'I mean, maybe it's just sort of John Wayne and Rambo culture, but I need to be self-sufficient. And when … my physical mechanism fails me, I am oftentimes just flooded with shame, self-hate and self-contempt' (LaForge 2025, p. 97). In addition, many found it really difficult to cope with friends and family who tried to be positive, when what they needed was someone to see their pain and to be able to accept that this was how things were. There is great solace in having someone who can quietly sit alongside you, but not try to change the situation. When such a person is lacking, it can be very frustrating. Chloe, in La Forge's study, said:

> If someone's like, 'things will get better …' just shut the fuck up, you have no way of knowing that […] the fluff talk can be so dangerous … And if you're seeing someone you care for, and they're telling you things that you know they can't back, it doesn't feel like a safe space anymore. It feels like, you know, handing someone a cupcake. And they don't want a cupcake. They just need you to sit there.
>
> (LaForge, 2025, p. 99)

So, as well as managing the responses of the health professionals and friends and family, and at the same time working hard to ensure their pain is taken seriously, people with persistent pain are finding out that they are the ones who need to ensure that they are keeping a close eye on all the different elements of their diagnosis journey and are beginning to become experts in navigating the system to get what they need to cope with their pain. This skill is increasingly required once they actually receive a diagnosis.

CHALLENGE 4: RECEIVING A DIAGNOSIS

Searching for an explanation for persistent pain does not always result in success. Indeed, over 40 per cent of adults who live with chronic pain have what is called diagnostic uncertainty (Neville et al., 2020). Not surprisingly, this uncertainty can be difficult to accept. Some researchers suggest that diagnostic uncertainty is linked to higher levels of anxiety and intensity of the pain experience (e.g., Serbic & Pincus, 2013). For some people, the diagnostic uncertainty leads them to carry on looking for an explanation by seeking more tests. This then becomes expensive for all concerned: for the person with the pain, who uses their time seeking tests, for the health professionals tasked with completing the tests, and for the health care system, in terms of the financial and time burden imposed.

Neville and colleagues (2020) interviewed health professionals about their experiences of diagnosing chronic pain. Although the focus of their study was on children diagnosed with chronic pain, the responses are just as relevant for adults. Health professionals were frustrated when they were unable to give certainty to patients. Physician 1, a woman who had been qualified for 28 years said:

> [...] as clinicians we are trained to find a problem, sort it out, give the medication or whatever it is, the treatment, and everybody's happy, everybody moves on, problem solved and that's it. But with chronic pain ... you can't do that, and so it's a completely different scenario, a different situation, and you just have to accept that sometimes there is no cause and there is no answer in terms of why, and whatever the situation is that you're faced with, that's the situation that you've got to deal with and try to improve.
>
> (Neville et al., 2020, p. 5)

So, many people, after having had multiple tests trying to get to the bottom of what is causing their persistent pain, never get a clear answer. For others, the receiving of a diagnosis of persistent pain may bring relief, but a diagnosis does not take away the pain. There is relief when finally, someone in authority provides a label for the pain. In addition, there is relief because someone believed that their pain was not all in their mind. Bruce and colleagues (2023), who interviewed Canadians about their pain journey, quoted one of their participants who described the difficulty of the journey to diagnosis.

Managing their knowledge that something really was wrong with them, while coping with test results that kept coming back negative, was exhausting. When the diagnosis came through, it was an important moment:

> The diagnosis was, was huge, it was a huge relief to finally hear, I mean like people would ask, you know, what's wrong, what's your diagnosis, nothing, I don't know, it's super frustrating to have nothing wrong with you but that's ridiculous... I know something is wrong.
>
> (Bruce et al., 2023, p. 5)

Similarly Karadag and colleagues (2025), who interviewed young adults about their coping strategies for their pain, also reported that their participants spoke of the relief and validation that a diagnosis offered them. For example, Chloe spoke of the uncertainty she faced while searching for her diagnosis: 'There was so many times where I would just doubt myself or invalidate myself because I didn't have a professional diagnosis'; while Theo highlighted the relief experienced on receiving a diagnosis: 'It was nice to know that there was a problem and I wasn't just making up the pain in my back' (Karadag et al., 2025, p. 7). This relief could be short lived. They now had a label, but they did not necessarily have an explanation, nor did they have a cure. The realisation that life had changed, and had changed for the foreseeable future, was not easy to take on board. Andersen and colleagues (2025), from Denmark, interviewed people who were living with pain to try to better understand the challenges they faced. For example, GR (a female diagnosed for 10 years) said: 'When you are in good health, you have a goal with your life and some routines ... and with a chronic illness, you have to rethink your life ... I wasn't prepared for how many things that would change in my life. No one told me about it.' This change that happened post-diagnosis was almost bittersweet because of the realisation that life would be different. For example, EV (a female diagnosed for 11 years) said: 'Receiving the diagnosis was like falling from a bench.

Suddenly I could not go on with things I did. And it took some time before I really understood that I actually was in a totally different situation.'

Keen and colleagues (2021, p. 746) based in London, also interviewed people about their pain. In their study, Participant 5 said:

> I experience it. I'm trying to understand what I'm supposed to be understanding, if that makes sense. Because I find that pain is an experience, it is not a concept. It is a concept for other people when they haven't got it, but it's not a concept for me, it is an experience.

Coming to terms with the diagnosis is therefore an important part of the process of learning to live with persistent pain.

CHALLENGE 5: ACCEPTING THE DIAGNOSIS

The act of being given a diagnosis can be described as a turning point. Although an individual may never discover the cause of their pain, the diagnosis of a chronic pain condition is confirmation that something really is wrong. However, it also brings another form of confirmation. The confirmation that they are now officially living with a long-term condition. This may not be welcome news and is likely to require some adjustment.

There is a model that was developed by Ellis-Hill and colleagues (2008) that can be useful when people are coming to terms with their diagnosis. The Life Thread model was originally developed to help understand the experience of identity change following an acquired disability. In the original paper that was published by Ellis-Hill and colleagues (2008), the authors focused on the impact of the experience of having a stroke. However, when I worked in practice with people who were living with all different types of persistent pain, I found that this model was a useful tool to help people move towards acceptance.

The Life Thread model recognises that as humans we are natural storytellers. We have a story ready to hand whenever someone asks us about ourselves. That life story (also known as a 'narrative thread') is a weaving together of all our experiences, as well as our interpretations of those experiences. Over time, as the story we tell is repeated, the weaving becomes strong and coherent and can be thought of as a thick thread made up of many thinner threads.

When we receive our diagnosis of persistent pain it can be experienced as a shock to our life story (narrative thread). Our strong rope that we have woven together over time is suddenly cut. Some threads are cut through cleanly by the diagnosis, others are frayed, some stay strong. It is unlikely that the clean-cut threads will mend, though some of the threads with frayed ends may be able to be woven back together. Threads that are woven back together can represent new ways of coping. For example, I worked with a person who used to ride horses and enjoyed competing in showjumping events. Their persistent pain made it very difficult for them to ride their horses. But they discovered that they could tolerate sitting sidesaddle. This opened up an opportunity for them to carry on riding their horses and they were also able to compete in dressage competitions. So, although they were no longer able to ride their horses in the way they had become used to, they found a new way to carry on with their beloved hobby. Applying the model, this person had found some brand new threads that they were able to weave into their rope. Their new rope looked similar, but was slightly different, symbolising new ways of doing old things.

The Life Thread model helped the people with whom I worked to begin to see what had happened to them in a different light. Their life did not stop, it continued to grow and change. We can forget that our lives are always changing as things around us change, as we change. Often these changes are more subtle than the diagnosis of a long-term condition. The person I was a year ago, is a very different person to who I am now. I have learned new things. I have experienced challenges (some of which I have overcome), all of which have changed me. The difference with a health condition is that it can be less subtle and gives us a more obvious knock to our life story.

So some threads are left untied and others are woven together in new ways. As this happens, we begin to reach a level of acceptance or adjustment. Chloe, in the study by Karadag and colleagues (2025, p. 11), said she had 'learned to adapt things a bit better, umm, so that I can still take part in things that I like doing'. Similarly, in the same study, Kelvin said: 'It's not where the world ends … basically, you have to adjust to lifestyle you know.' The importance of coming to terms with, of accepting, the diagnosis was summarised by one of the participants in the study by Bruce and colleagues (2023, p. 6):

> If you are not accepting, if you are constantly fighting against it and try to figure out what's wrong or how do we turn this off, like it's like beating your head against a brick wall as opposed to learning, finding ways to cope with it. Coping cannot start until you accept it.

CHALLENGE 6: BECOMING YOUR OWN PAIN EXPERT

The process of learning to cope with and accept the diagnosis, while also managing their own response and the responses of others, in effect teaches people living with persistent pain to become their own pain expert. For example, Dupont and colleagues (2025), based in Germany, interviewed people living with persistent pain as well as GPs. The people living with pain recognised that they had a responsibility to play an active role in interactions with the GPs. They said that treatment could not be something done by the GP *to* them, but had to be something in which they were actively involved. This was summarised by Participant 22 who said: 'I am always the main actor, it is up to me whether I get back on my feet or not' (Dupont et al., 2025, p. 7). This was a perspective that was also held by the GPs, though when I read between the lines in this paper, it seemed to me that, rather than seeing themselves working together with people in pain, the GPs saw themselves as experts telling people in pain what to do and expecting the person in pain to do their bit. Two quotes from

GPs (Dupont et al., 2025) highlight their underlying expectation that patients should do as they are told:

> For example, he has to do his exercises for lumbar and spine problems, we prescribe physiotherapy for him and then he doesn't do his exercises and then he comes to me and says the pain isn't getting any better. [GP 21]

> I can suggest it [...] but then there is usually no willingness on the other side. And then I know that it will not be carried out properly. [...] but the patient has to initiate it and then it happens quite well. [GP 06]

This second quote is to my eyes quite telling. If a patient initiates it, 'it happens quite well'. If the GP suggests it, there is no willingness on the other side. Very few of us like being told what to do. But if we are consulted and listened to, and our life context is taken into account when treatment is being planned, and if we have played an active role in the process, then of course we are more likely to do whatever the recommendation is.

In short, the process of navigating the health system teaches people that they need to take responsibility and coordinate the care they need. Hadi and colleagues (2017) showed that people living with persistent pain felt that GPs tended to prescribe medication, regardless of whether the person with pain was gaining any benefit. For example, Participant 9 in their study said: 'According to them [GPs] all they could do was give me paracetamol, and the best was co-codamol' (Hadi et al., 2017, p. 5). Others felt they were sent for physiotherapy because it what was done, rather than what was necessarily needed. Participant 4 said: 'I think the GP finds it an easy ... she doesn't know ... it's the easy answer to shove you to the physio and let them have a look at you and then see what bounces back out of that' (Hadi et al., 2017, p. 4). Similarly, Shakespeare (2021, p. 118) wrote:

> I discovered recently that the painkillers I have been taking since I became paralysed on 20 August 2008 have damaging effects

> on concentration and memory. Interacting with normal ageing the result is that I become forgetful, my academic work suffers. This is unacceptable to me, but so is the pain I get if I stop taking the tablets.

There is clearly a need for people living with persistent pain to play an active role in their own care. But they can only do this if the health professionals take them seriously and recognise that people who live with pain come with self-knowledge and expertise in their experiences and their life context. A willingness to work together to join the expertise of the person with pain and that of the person who treats pain will result in more holistic care.

SO, WHAT IS IT LIKE TO LIVE WITH PERSISTENT PAIN?

As well as coping with their pain, the person in pain has to cope with the impact of their pain. The impact takes many forms. Managing other people's responses to your pain is one of the biggest challenges of the pain experience. The next chapter focuses on why it is so hard to explain persistent pain to someone else.

FURTHER RESOURCES

Useful articles

BBC article: The curse of people who never feel pain. https://www.bbc.com/future/article/20170426-the-people-who-never-feel-any-pain [accessed 21 February 2026].

NBC article: How one man's mutant DNA may help end the deadly opioid crisis. https://www.nbcnews.com/mach/science/how-one-man-s-mutant-dna-may-help-end-deadly-ncna788181 [accessed 21 February 2026].

NHS. How to get help for your pain. https://www.nhs.uk/live-well/pain/how-to-get-nhs-help-for-your-pain/.

Useful organisations

Action on Pain: Lobbies national and local politicians about the provision of pain services and provides support and advice for people who are affected by persistent pain. https://action-on-pain.co.uk/

Contact: A charity for families with disabled children. It has some information on CIP, written by Professor Geoff Woods, an expert in CIP. https://contact.org.uk/conditions/congenital-insensitivityindifference-to-pain/ [accessed 21 February 2026].

Pain Concern: Produces information on pain, provides support to people with pain and those who care for them, raises awareness, and campaigns to improve the provision of pain management services. https://painconcern.org.uk/#.

Pain Toolkit: Developed by Pete Moore to help people with persistent pain self-manage. https://www.paintoolkit.org/.

Useful books

Peacock, S. (2018). *Managing chronic pain in the family: Help for all the family*. Ann Jaloba Publishing

Peacock, S. (2016). *Sleeping with pain: Strategies for a restful night from pain management*. Ann Jaloba Publishing.

REFERENCES

Andersen, A.H., Hvidt, E.A., Huniche, L., et al. (2025). Why we suffer? Existential challenges of patients with chronic illness: A Kierkegaardian inspired interpretative phenomenological analysis. *Journal of Humanistic Psychology*, 65(5), 969–996.

BBC (2017) The curse of the people who never feel pain. https://www.bbc.co.uk/future/article/20170426-the-people-who-never-feel-any-pain [accessed 7 August 2025].

Bruce, M., Lopatina, E., Hodge, J., et al. (2023). Understanding the chronic pain journey and coping strategies that patients use to manage their chronic pain: A qualitative patient-led, Canadian study. *BMJ Open*, 13, e072048. doi: 10.1136/bmjopen-2023-072048.

Clarke, A., Anthony. G., Gray, D., et al. (2012). 'I feel so stupid because I can't give a proper answer ...': How older adults describe chronic pain. A qualitative study. *BMC Geriatrics*, 12: 78.

Corkhill, B. (2021). Pain signals and other bad language. In P. Wemyss-Gorman (ed.), *Innovative approaches to chronic pain: Understanding the experience of pain and suffering and the role of healing*. Jessica Kingsley Publishers.

Costa, N., Butler, P., Dillon, M., et al. (2023). 'I felt uncertain about my whole future': A qualitative investigation of people's experiences of navigating uncertainty when seeking care for their low back pain. *Pain*, 164, 2749–2758.

De Ruddere, L. and Craig, K.D. (2016). Understanding stigma and chronic pain: A state-of-the-art review. *Pain*, 157(8), 1607–1610.

De Ruddere, L., Goubert, L., Vervoot, T. et al. (2012). We discount the pain of others when pain has no medical explanation. *The Journal of Pain*, 13(12), 1198–1205.

Drissi, I., Woods, W.A., and Woods, C.G. (2020). Understanding the genetic basis of congenital insensitivity to pain. *British Medical Bulletin*, 133, 65–78.

Dupont, D., Brinkmöller, S., Carter, S., et al. (2025). Exploring physician and patient perspectives on expectations and role models towards chronic pain treatment in general practice: A qualitative cross-sectional study. *Healthcare*, 13, 187. https://doi.org/10.3390/healthcare13020187.

Ellis-Hill, C., Payne, S., and Ward, C. (2008). Using stroke to explore the Life Thread model: An alternative approach to understanding rehabilitation following an acquired disability. *Disability and Rehabilitation*, 30(2), 150–159.

Hadi, M.A., Alldred, D.P., Briggs, M., et al. (2017). 'Treated as a number, not treated as a person': A qualitative exploration of the perceived barriers to effective pain management of patients with chronic pain. *BMJ Open*, 7, e016454.

Itmaiza, M.N., Skafi, A.J., Adawi, A.A., et al. (2025). First instance of pain in congenital pan insensitivity with anhidrosis. *Clinical Neurology and Neurosurgery*, 249, 108775. https://doi.org/10.1016/j.clineuro.2025.108775.

Kang, Y., Trewern, L., Jackman, J., et al. (2023). Chronic pain: Definitions and diagnosis. *BMJ*, 381, e076036.

Karadag, P., Taylor, J., and Burton, A. (2025). Self-management and coping in young adults with chronic pain: A reflexive thematic analysis. *Journal of Health Psychology*. doi: 10.1177/13591053251344236.

Keen, S., Lomeli-Rodriguez, M., and C de C Williams, A. (2021). Exploring how people with chronic pain understand their pain: A qualitative study. *Scandinavian Journal of Pain*, 21(4), 743–753.

King's Fund (2025). https://www.kingsfund.org.uk/insight-and-analysis/data-and-charts/waiting-times-non-urgent-treatment#how-long-are-the-waiting-lists-for-different-specialties? [accessed 27 December 2025].

LaForge, K. (2025). 'Just because I'm smiling doesn't mean I'm not in pain': Navigating the layered stigma of chronic pain and suicidality in social worlds. *Health Sociology Review*, 34(1), 92–107. https://doi.org/10.1080/14461242.2024.2398250.

Liddy, C., Cooper, L., Bellingham, G., et al. (2024). Patient-reported wait times and the impact of living with chronic pain on their quality of life: A waiting room survey in chronic pain clinics in Ontario, Manitoba and Quebec. *Canadian Journal of Pain*, 8(1), 2345612. https://doi.org/10.1080/24740527.2024.2345612.

Lynch, M.E., Campbell, F., Clark, A.J., et al. (2008). A systematic review of the effect of waiting for treatment for chronic pain. *Pain*, 136, 97–116.

McCaffery, M. (1968). *Nursing practice theories related to cognition, bodily pain, and man-environment interactions*. University of Los Angeles.

Neville, A., Noel, M., Clinch, J., et al. (2020). 'Drawing a line in the sand': Physician diagnostic uncertainty in paediatric chronic pain. *European Journal of Pain*, 25(2), 430–441. https://doi.org/10.1002/ejp.1682

Rodham, K. (2015). *Learning to cope with CRPS/RSD: Putting life first and pain second*. Singing Dragon.

Schon, K.R., Parker, A.P.J,. and Woods, C.G. (2020). Congenital insensitivity to pain overview. In M.P. Adam, J. Feldman, G.M. Mirzaa, et al. (eds), *GeneReviews® [Internet]*. University of Washington, Seattle; 1993–202.

Serbic, D. and Pincus, T. (2013). Chasing the ghosts: The impact of diagnostic labelling on self-management and pain-related guilt in chronic low back pain patients. *Journal of Pain Management*, 1(6), 25–35.

Shakespeare, T. (2021). 'This is going to hurt me more than it hurts you': The problem of pain. In P. Wemyss-Gorman (ed.), *Innovative approaches to chronic pain: Understanding the experience of pain and suffering and the role of healing*. Jessica Kingsley Publishers.

Upshur, C.C., Bacigalupe, G., and Luckmann, R. (2010). 'They don't want anything to do with you': Patient views of primary care management of chronic pain. *Pain Medicine*, 11, 1791–1798.

Van Hout, F., Van Rooden, A., and Slatman, J. (2023). Chronicling the chronic: Narrating the meaninglessness of chronic pain. *Medical Humanities*, 49, 1–8.

3

WHY IS IT SO HARD TO EXPLAIN PERSISTENT PAIN TO SOMEONE ELSE?

INTRODUCTION

Shakespeare (2021, p. 112), wrote 'nothing is as absorbing as pain, but nothing is as boring as someone else's pain. Even more boring than someone else's holiday photographs'. This quote is not by the Shakespeare who wrote all those plays (after all, photographs were not around in the 1500s!), but is from Tom Shakespeare, a professor of disability research and a campaigner for disability rights. He also lives with persistent pain. This quote sums up the difficulty facing those who live with persistent pain have in explaining what their experience is like. He goes on to write that, even though we all feel pain, understanding the pain of another person is very difficult. Pain is a sensation and so is not easy to put into words. We expect pain to be fixable. When someone's pain cannot be fixed, people without pain struggle to understand what the person in pain is going through. And because people do not understand, it is easy for them to dismiss another person's pain. As Shakespeare says, nothing is as boring as someone else's pain.

If you are not someone who is living with persistent pain, take a moment to think about the last time you experienced pain. Maybe you broke a bone, maybe you overdid the gardening, maybe you

DOI: 10.4324/9781003649854-3

fell over and picked up some bumps and bruises, maybe you had toothache. The cause of the pain in this example is irrelevant. What is important is the pain you experienced and how you explained your pain experience to someone else. How easy was it to share your experience? Did you think the other person really understood just how much pain you were in at that time? What words did you use to describe your pain? Was explaining what the pain was like easier than saying what the pain was? The quote from a Canadian participant in a study reported by Bruce and colleagues (2023, p. 4) summarises the difficulty we face when trying to explain our pain to others: 'I sure wish we could change bodies for about five minutes so that you could better understand exactly where I am coming from.'

In 1968, Margo McCaffery said that, since we could not objectively measure pain, we had to rely on the person experiencing the pain to tell us what it was like. In short, McCaffery said that pain was whatever that person who had the pain said it was. She argued that we had to take on trust what the person was telling us. Indeed, McCaffery is remembered by Pasero (2018) as being someone who would call people out who did not take on trust what people in pain said they were experiencing. Pasero (2018, p. 90) recalls Margo as being:

> [...] outspoken, fearless, and unapologetic when confronting misconceptions and bias against people with pain [...] she stood up at a national pain conference to ask a well credentialed speaker to provide references for his particularly disrespectful and inaccurate statements about people with pain.

However, it turns out that we are not always so good at explaining our pain. This is something which is explored in a paper by Charles Djordjevic (2023), in which he argues that 'pain cannot (just) be whatever the person says'. Djordjevic shares McCaffery's original outrage about the under-treatment of pain but also suggests that 'our continued inability to deal humanely with pain suggests we have missed something crucial about it' (Djordjevic, 2023, p. 2). In his paper, Djordjevic explores the need to work with the person in pain to understand their context, their needs, and, sometimes, to help them finds ways to express their pain. And so he argues that, if a health professional has helped the person to find a way of expressing their pain, technically the pain becomes what the person in pain and the health professional together say it is. The paper is a really interesting exploration of how we try to explain our pain. And that is really the essence of this chapter. How do we explain pain to others?

There are many challenges that can get in the way of our ability to trust what another person says about their pain. These may include that person's ability to say how they are feeling. After all, not everyone is able to find the words to share their experience. Maybe we are influenced by a person's race, gender, socioeconomic status, education level, and so forth. These biases and prejudices influence how we perceive others. Some studies have even shown that how believable you are, depends on how likeable you are. It turns out it is not so easy to explain your experience of persistent pain to someone else. So perhaps we need to start with exploring how we measure pain.

MEASURING PAIN

In Chapter 1, I explained how persistent or chronic pain is defined. You will remember that this is usually described as being defined by time, in that if the pain has lasted for three months or more, it is considered to be persistent (chronic) pain (Kang et al., 2023; Nicholas et al., 2019). In this chapter, I want to think a little bit more about the way in which we measure pain and the problems of measuring something that is an internal individual experience.

Elaine Scarry (1985) wrote that 'physical pain has no voice' and 'comes unsharably into our midst as at once that which cannot be denied and that which cannot be confirmed'. This, I think, captures a huge challenge facing people who live with pain, for health professionals who are trying to help those who live with pain, and for those who want to research the pain experience. Pain is a sensation. It is not visible, and it is not something that can be reliably measured. In Chapter 1, I noted that our 'pain detection system' sends messages to our brain – so maybe we could measure the activity of the detection system? However, the pain detection system in and of itself is not sufficient to bring about the experience of pain. Our brain is also involved. It receives the messages and then works out whether or not the messages equal pain. So, if something cannot be reliably measured, as Scarry (1985) noted, it can neither be denied nor confirmed. This is why McCaffery's work was so important in reminding health professionals that the person who was experiencing the pain was, in effect, the pain expert.

Of course, this has not stopped us from trying to measure pain. Pain is usually measured using rating scales. This involves the person who says they are experiencing pain being asked to rate their pain (usually on a scale of zero to ten, where ten is the worst pain imaginable and zero is no pain). Although this seems to be a straightforward task, choosing a number to represent the experience of your chronic pain is not so easy. For a pain that is fleeting (e.g., stubbing your toe), arguably choosing a number is fairly simple. Following the initial bump, there is a short gap and then suddenly the pain explodes. You might be hopping around (possibly swearing – see Chapter 5), and you could easily say that the pain is a 'ten'. Relatively quickly though, the pain lessens and moves from sharp to throbbing and then fades. In line with this, your scores would also drop. This is because scales are typically designed to measure pain intensity.

The persistent pain experience is different. It is not just about the pain intensity. This difference was explored by Hush and colleagues (2009) who ran a series of groups with 36 adults who had either recovered from or were still experiencing back pain. These people were asked about their experiences of recovery and what recovery meant to them. They were also asked to comment on the 'zero to ten' measure of pain intensity and a questionnaire designed to identify the impact of low back pain on many different aspects of daily living. The groups were asked how meaningful the two measures were in terms of capturing changes in their condition. Group members said that it was not easy to say if someone was recovered or unrecovered. Indeed, when Hush and colleagues (2009) looked at the pain scores group members had chosen, they found that these did not necessarily tally with whether they had described themselves as recovered or unrecovered. Half of the group who decided they could be classified as 'recovered' scored between 1 and 3 out of 10 on the pain rating scale. Similarly, more than half of those in the 'unrecovered' group had low back pain scores of 3 or less. In the discussions, group members made it clear that pain was a factor in their recovery. For example, a participant said: 'I'd know when I'm better when I can put on my shoes and socks without my back hurting, and not actually [have to] sit down and think "Oh here we go".' However, an absence of pain was not a reliable indicator of complete recovery. By way of example, one participant said: 'I'm still careful about some things I do … being careful just managing the potential for pain, because I don't have back pain, but I am careful about what I do' (Hush and colleagues 2009, p. 127). Recovery was all about noticing improved performance in their daily activities: 'I can tell when it's better … when you feel like you're walking taller and your neck and everything feels softer.' These findings were of interest because they showed that the relationship between the pain scores and the recovery status of the individuals was less clear than had previously been assumed. A low pain score was found in both those who considered themselves 'recovered' and those who said they were 'unrecovered'. The study by Hush and colleagues (2009) highlights the importance of remembering to ask the patient what is important to them.

Similarly, Yorkston and colleagues (2010) wanted to better understand how patients spoke to health professionals about their pain. They recruited 23 adults who were living with persistent pain and put them into five groups to explore a range of issues (for example: How has pain affected your daily activities? What has been the greatest impact of pain on your life?) as well as exploring how they spoke with the doctors about their pain. The participants discussed which words they used when talking about pain. Some focused on describing the qualities of their pain (throbbing, numb, sharp), or trying to explain what it was like (e.g., sitting on razor blades, a bad toothache). Others talked about the timing of their pain; for some it was constant, for others it caught them by surprise. One person mentioned really liking the kinds of scales that listed lots of words for pain, but then said that even though this was useful 'it doesn't really get to the heart of the matter'.

In terms of using the rating scale, giving numbers to pain from 0 to 10 was described as very difficult for a range of reasons. People found 0 and 10 were relatively straightforward, either there was no pain or there were huge amounts of pain; but they found using the numbers in between really difficult. One person said: 'I think everyone experiences pain differently'; and another said: 'What's a 4 to me might be an 8 to somebody else or might be a 1 to somebody else.' Still others made the point that when you live with persistent pain, you are never without pain. One person suggested that, for her, a score of 4 was what she called her normal level of pain. This meant that the numbers available to this person to record their pain were 4 and upwards. She could not make use of the whole scale. In the way that 0 is the baseline score for someone who lives without persistent pain, for this participant, 4 equated to her baseline.

Participants in this study were also asked whether there were questions that they wished their health professionals would ask them. Responses to this question highlighted a wish that health professionals would show interest in understanding just how living with persistent pain impacts on life. These included: 'What is pain preventing you from doing?' and 'How long does it take you to get up and ready for the day?'. They also wanted to be included in discussions about pain management and to have a greater focus on *how* they were coping, rather than the tools and techniques for coping. They wanted to be asked: 'What are you doing to take care of yourself?' and 'What do you do to make yourself feel better?' and 'What triggers your pain?' One participant summed this up in the following quote: 'They speak to me less about what I can do to make myself feel better and more about what is the function, what is the angle of your leg and how can we increase your baclofen [medicine]' (Yorkston et al., 2010, p. 248). This study shows that persistent pain is complex – it is not just about pain intensity – and it is also an individual experience. For both these reasons, pain rating scales are not likely to fully capture the experience of living with persistent pain. People who live with persistent pain know this, and this research shows that they want health professionals, as a minimum, to look beyond the rating scales.

IF SCALES ARE NOT A GOOD FIT, HOW ELSE MIGHT WE HELP PEOPLE TO COMMUNICATE THEIR PERSISTENT PAIN EXPERIENCE?

Given the complexity of the persistent pain experience, researchers and practitioners have explored using other techniques. For example, Dr Adrianna Loduca in Brazil developed the Pain Portrait. I consider myself very lucky to have met Adrianna. I was awarded some funding from the University of Bath when I worked there to cover the costs of a visit to the hospital in São Paulo, Brazil, where Adrianna worked. As well as being able to sit in on her pain clinics, I was also able to observe a pain management group and learn about the Pain Portrait work Loduca and her colleagues had been using (see Loduca et al., 2014, for an overview of this work). The Pain Portrait work was developed by the Brazilian pain management team who wanted to find a way to open up conversations with their patients about their pain. They asked their patients to draw their pain. Once the drawing was complete, they asked a series of questions about the drawing. As well as asking the patients to talk through their drawing, they also asked whether they could give their pain a name. Some patients gave their pain a human name, some named the pain after the most prominent symptom they were experiencing during the interview. Some simply called their pain 'pain'. They were also asked how old the pain was. The question was not about how long they had lived with pain, but how old the pain was. I remember when one patient who had lived with pain for a couple of years said that their pain was an old pain; a pain in its 70s. They found that patients were better able to express their pain experiences and (with echoes of McCaffery's work) highlighted the importance of listening to patients' own experiences of their pain. This process helped the patients find a way to describe their pain. And because the person with pain and the health professional sat side by side to look together at the pain portrait, it was clear that they were working together to find a way to live well in spite of the persistent pain. The relationship dynamic changed from 'expert' and 'patient' to collaborators.

In Australia, a different creative approach has been explored by Drogemuller and colleagues (2025). They developed a machine that enabled people to design a 3D object that represented their pain. The intention was to turn an internal experience into an external object. The machine invited participants to change the shape of a sphere that was on the screen so that it could represent their personal pain experience. There were four sliding buttons which could be used to change the shape (e.g., adding spikes or creating holes). Once a person had finished adapting the shape, they were asked to describe the painful experience that their object represented. After this, the participants could print their pain objects in 3D (one for them and one for the researchers). Through holding the pain objects, people could physically experience the representation of another person's pain. To me, this is a high-tech version of the Pain Portrait study. Instead of using drawing, it uses technology and invites people to find a way to represent their pain and make the invisible visible. Both approaches help the person in pain, who may be struggling to find the words to explain their pain, to create something that captures their experience more fully than a simple score of 1 to 10. The object or image itself opens up conversations about their pain experience.

DO WE HAVE THE SAME UNDERSTANDING OF THE WORDS USED TO DESCRIBE PAIN?

As noted at the end of the last paragraph, it can be a struggle to find the right words to explain what living with chronic pain is like. This struggle can be made harder if the words chosen are not understood in the way they are meant. After all, words used to describe pain are not useful in medical consultations if the health professional and the person in pain understand them in different ways (see Kenny et al., 2006). This again, highlights the importance of McCaffery's statement about pain being whatever the person experiencing it says it is. In other words, health professionals need to make sure that they have the same understanding of what the person in pain is saying about their pain.

As an aside, this reminds me of the way emergency department staff respond in the United Kingdom when they hear that a farmer is being brought in by ambulance. Having watched many of the programmes that follow emergency department staff or paramedics, I have learned that if a farmer agrees to be brought in to a hospital, the assumption of the health professionals is that the farmer will likely be very seriously injured and, at the same time, will be playing down their injuries so they can get back to work as soon as possible. There is an understanding that when a farmer says something hurts a bit, it is quite likely that they are understating their experience. So, when McCaffery said that pain is whatever the person experiencing it says it is, the health professional has a responsibility to double check that what the person says is properly understood. In short, checking our understanding of the words chosen when people are describing their pain experience is important. But this is only part of the story, because we need to be wise to the fact that our understanding of what people are saying is influenced by a range of other factors.

DO WE MAKE ASSUMPTIONS ABOUT HOW PEOPLE FROM DIFFERENT CULTURAL AND ETHNIC GROUPS EXPERIENCE PAIN?

In their review of influences on chronic pain, Maly and Vallerand (2018) note that racism in health care practice has long been an issue. Similarly, Schubiner and colleagues (2023, p. 1729) note that:

> Black Americans are less likely to be screened for pain, referred for pain management, and adequately treated than White Americans. These health care inequities are built upon historically rooted and unfortunately persistent beliefs that Black people feel less pain than White people – harmful myths that have persisted since slavery. We propose that racism is a key determinant of the disproportionate burden of severe pain among Black Americans.

Ghoshal and colleagues (2023), quoting Byrd and Clayton (2001) note that racism in medicine can be seen as far back in time as the ancient Greeks, who viewed all slaves as inferior and less intelligent. Similarly, they mention a second-century Roman doctor called Galen who viewed White people as superior to non-White people. This 'othering' has continued through time and has led to horrendous treatment of, and attitudes towards, non-White people, which continues today. Ghoshal and colleagues (2023), writing in the United States, note that implicit bias continues to exert a negative influence on the care received by, and outcomes of, people from minority ethnic groups. For example, Strand and colleagues (2021) list a depressing number of studies highlighting the bias against Black people in the American health system. They share research that shows doctors consider White patients more cooperative medically than Black patients (Oliver et al., 2014); that Black patients are less likely to be prescribed opioids for acute pain than White patients (Jarman et al., 2022; Mills et al., 2011); and that White medical trainees can believe that Black patients feel less pain, which leads to inaccurate diagnoses and treatment plans (Hoffman et al., 2016).

Leach and colleagues (2024), who were mentioned briefly in Chapter 1, reviewed papers that focused on access to chronic pain services for adults from minority ethnic groups in the United Kingdom. They note that the NHS guidance states that all services should support equality and deliver services that meet the needs of patients, including those from minority ethnic groups. However, their review failed to find any studies that had tried to explore the ethnic profile of people accessing pain services. Neither were there any that specifically assessed ethnic disparities within chronic pain services. This failure to collect and report accurate ethnicity records means we do not currently know how many people from minority ethnic groups are able to access this support. Given that we know that, in the United Kingdom, self-reported chronic pain is more common among people from minority ethnic groups compared to White ethnic groups (see Allison, et al., 2002; Choudhury et al., 2013; Palmer et al., 2007), it is important that this data is collected. Leach and colleagues (2024,

p. 3505) conclude: 'This future work is essential in identifying health-care disparity issues for adults from minority ethnic groups that can be addressed by chronic pain services to remove such inequalities.'

A person's ethnicity has also been shown to impact on whether or not they are considered to be in real pain or faking pain (see the review by Lin and colleagues (2023) of 40 experimental studies and the paper by Mende-Siedlecki and colleagues, 2021). Paige-Lloyd and colleagues (2022) designed a series of studies where participants were asked to view videos or pictures of Black and White individuals experiencing actual pain or faking pain. Participants had to say whether the pain was real or fake. Across all six studies, the people viewing the videos and images struggled to tell the difference between real and fake expressions for Black compared to White people. This was true for both medical providers and people from the general population. In other words, this study showed that there was consistent inaccuracy in reading Black people's pain. Black people's pain was judged and treated less accurately than that of White people.

So we know that non-White groups have been treated very badly by health care systems. These experiences continue. This means accessing health care when you live with chronic pain, and you are not White, is even harder. We also know that when you do access it, you are more likely to receive a poorer service. As noted by Leach and colleagues (2024) we need to do better at collecting data in order to evidence this disparity properly so that we can make sure equality of access is central to pain services.

DO WE MAKE ASSUMPTIONS ABOUT HOW GENDER INFLUENCES THE PAIN EXPERIENCE AND DOES THIS THEN IMPACT ON WHETHER AND HOW AN EXPLANATION OF PAIN IS HEARD?

It is well established that gender can impact on how health professionals assess and manage pain. Patrick-Smith and Bull (2024) explain that gender bias can result from stereotyping, where you are treated differently in a clinically unjustified way because of your gender. It can also happen via something called 'gender blindness', which is what happens when clinically important differences between the genders are overlooked. For example, Hoffman and Tarzian (2001) concluded that women were more likely to try to get help for chronic pain, but they were also likely to be inadequately treated. They suggested that health professionals were more likely to discount women's verbal pain reports: 'while men may be seen as forceful or aggressive, women are perceived as hysterical for the same behaviour' (Hoffman and Tarzian, 2001, p. 20). In other words, because women were more likely to express their feelings when reporting pain, they were more likely than men to have their symptoms linked to emotional factors. This then resulted in their pain either not being properly diagnosed or being undertreated.

Twenty-three years on from the Hoffman and Tarzian (2001) study, Patrick-Smith and Bull (2024) reviewed the literature on medical student perceptions of gender and pain. They found that gender was still influencing student perceptions of patient pain. Women were generally considered to be more pain sensitive than men, were regarded as being more distressed, and thought to be more inclined to exaggerate the level of pain they were in. It is worth pointing out that Patrick-Smith and Bull (2024) highlighted that most of the studies they reviewed were simulations, so it is not clear whether the perceptions would be the same in real-life interactions. Nevertheless, this is a concerning finding.

Seventy different studies focusing on women's experience of persistent pain were reviewed by Biring and colleagues (2025). They showed that women faced a dual burden when managing their pain alongside the demands of their lives. Parenting and caregiving made their pain worse (e.g., Johnson et al., 2024; Rice et al., 2024). One participant in a study by Evans and De Souza (2008) said 'looking after children was the hardest part of pain'. A key challenge mentioned by the women in these studies was the invisibility of their pain and the impact this had on seeking help and understanding. For example, a participant in a study by Wuytack and Miller (2011,

p. 6) spoke about their persistent pain. She said: 'They don't understand it because they don't see it [...] I used to give a lot of explanation, but now I can't be bothered any more. There are very few people who understand it.' Similarly, Brown and colleagues (2024) ran focus groups with 57 women who were living with bladder pain and who had experienced interactions with health professionals who did not believe them, or who dismissed their pain. They also spoke of the invisibility of their pain and how health professionals would say that they 'looked fine' to them. Because of how they appeared to the health professionals, some women spoke of how they felt that their pain was belittled. They shared their experiences of being told that they were highly strung, overly anxious, and that they should be more positive. In other words, the unspoken suggestion being that they were the cause of their own pain. The most common experience shared was that of struggling to make other people understand that their condition was real and valid. This was bad enough if the disbelief came from friends and employers, but was much worse when health professionals dismissed their experience. Biring and colleagues (2025, p. 40) reported women feeling 'dismissed, rejected, disbelieved and ignored' by health professionals. One participant in a study by Reibel and Pearson (2017) said that their rheumatologist told her that he knew what fibromyalgia was, but that he did not believe in it. Another woman in a study by Johnson and colleagues (2024) said that a health professional told her that women often exaggerated pain. These negative experiences inevitably shape participants' subsequent health-seeking behaviour, outlook, and wellbeing.

DOES HOW LIKEABLE SOMEONE IS IMPACT ON HOW THEIR PAIN IS PERCEIVED?

De Ruddere and colleagues (e.g., 2011, 2012, 2013, 2014) have written a series of papers about how people in pain are perceived. They developed a series of vignettes (mini-case studies), which they showed to participants. The vignettes either described the presence or absence of medical evidence for the pain reported by the person in pain. First photos were looked at, then videos were viewed. The person featured then had their pain rated by the participant. Some vignettes showed people in obvious pain, others expressed low-level pain. People who viewed the vignettes were less inclined to be sympathetic when medical evidence for the pain was absent (De Ruddere et al., 2013). Worse though was that participants were less likely to want to help the person in a vignette if there was no medical evidence for the pain, even if the person in the vignette was clearly in a lot of pain. The people in this study were drawn from the general population. In other words, they could be our family, our friends, and our colleagues. They are the people we would turn to if we were experiencing persistent chronic pain. If our pain was persistent but there was no medical evidence to explain it, how confident are we that our friends, family, and colleagues would be sympathetic? Remember Tom Shakespeare's quote about how other people's pain is more boring than other people's holiday photographs? Remember too that the 'general population' is also 'us'. You and me. How confident are you that you would be sympathetic to friends, family, and colleagues living with persistent pain?

The way in which health professionals react to people living with persistent pain has also been explored by De Ruddere and colleagues (2014). Using a similar vignette, the health professionals were asked to estimate, among other things, the amount of pain the person in the vignette was experiencing and their own sympathy for the person in pain. The findings were the same. Where medical evidence for the pain was absent, ratings on all measures were lower. The level of pain displayed in the vignette did not influence the ratings, other than to increase suspicion that the person in pain might be exaggerating. So, health professionals also disregard the information given by the person in pain. McCaffery's statement – that pain is whatever a person in pain says it is – is ignored. Worse still, another study completed by the team (De Ruddere et al., 2011), explored whether how likeable a person was perceived to be would influence how seriously their pain was taken. Although the team again relied on vignettes (which remove face-to-face cues, interactions, and rapport building), they found that patients who were not liked were thought to be in less pain than those who were liked. It is clear, then, that we must all become more aware of our own potential bias. Indeed, the title of the paper by De Ruddere and colleagues (2011) is telling: 'When you dislike patients, pain is taken less seriously.' Obviously there were limitations to the study but nonetheless it provides a thought-provoking insight into the influence of unconscious bias and how this could impact on the care offered to people living with persistent pain.

DOES USING METAPHORS HELP TO COMMUNICATE PAIN?

Stephen Loftus (2011, p. 218) argues that metaphors 'profoundly shape the way the general population, as well as doctors conceptualise their health problems'. For example, in the West, the dominant metaphor for the body is as a machine. Loftus (2011) notes that this metaphor can work well. After all, when things go wrong with our body, we take it to a health professional to be fixed in the same way that we would take our car to a garage. The problem is that the metaphor of 'body as machine' leads people to expect 'that malfunctions' can be 'fixed'. In the context of persistent pain, if the 'body as machine' metaphor continues to be used, patients may 'come to believe that the "damage" they think must be causing their pain is continuing to do them more and more harm because that is what happens in machines that malfunction and are not repaired properly' (Loftus, 2011, p. 220). This, Loftus argues, is why persistent pain can be so frustrating for both the health professional and the person living with persistent pain: the metaphor is not adequate or appropriate.

Similarly, Jasmine Hearn and her team (2024) explored the metaphors used by people living with persistent pain. The seventy people who took part in the study were asked to complete a series of questionnaires and then they were asked a free text question: 'The pain feels like …'. They were invited to give as much detail as they wanted. The average length of time people in the study had lived with persistent pain was 14.5 years. The six most common conditions they were living with were arthritis, neuropathic pain, fibromyalgia, endometriosis, back pain, and complex regional pain syndrome. What was interesting about this study is the suggestion that people with different pain conditions used different kinds of pain metaphor. For example, people with arthritis used metaphors about physical damage ('it feels as though there should be a stake or a knife sticking in there'), while people with endometriosis used metaphors about pain being an evil thing that is causing the damage ('someone has a large roughly scrunched up ball of tin foil and wire in my belly and is twisting and turning it'). The team call for more work to be done that would help explore how useful these metaphors might be in helping to improve communication as well as understanding and empathy between patients, family, and, of course, health professionals.

SO, WHY IS IT SO HARD TO EXPLAIN PERSISTENT PAIN TO SOMEONE ELSE?

Pain is an individual experience. It is invisible and it is very hard to describe. This difficulty in explaining pain can bring shame and embarrassment to the person living with pain, as shown in this extract from an interview shared by Clarke and colleagues (2012, p. 4):

> Person with pain: 'I can't really explain to you how embarrassed I feel because really there isn't words to explain ...'
>
> Interviewer: 'Why would you feel embarrassed about it? It's an interesting term, embarrassment.'
>
> Person with pain: 'That I don't have the vocabulary and I haven't got the medical vocabulary. I don't have the jargon to explain what I'm feeling.' [Caucasian Male 9, aged 68, with foot pain]

We also know from the work of De Ruddere and colleagues, that people in pain need to perform in order to get the treatment they need, and they also need to be likeable. There are other factors that influence how people are seen and whether they are heard, with gender and race being two important challenges that influence the pain experiences of females and Non-White people who live with pain. Failure to understand the persistent myths surrounding the experience of pain leads to inadequate interactions with health professionals as well as negative treatment experiences. In a paper entitled: 'Your patient is in pain, here is how you respond', McCaffery and Robinson (2002, p. 38) said 'Expecting a patient to "act" like he's in pain is one of the most common reasons why nurses don't treat pain'. Having established the reasons why it is so hard to explain persistent pain to someone else, in the next chapter, I focus on why it is so hard to manage your own pain.

FURTHER RESOURCES

For a slightly sweary review of pain rating scales, you could read this light-hearted, but also serious, blog post. https://hyperboleandahalf.blogspot.com/2010/02/boyfriend-doesnt-have-ebola-probably.html [accessed 14 September 2025].

Flippin pain: Public health campaign with a clear goal: to change the way we think about, talk about, and treat persistent pain. https://www.flippinpain.co.uk/resources/.

Moseley's how to explain pain video: https://youtu.be/jIsF8CXouk8?feature=shared.

For an insight into the gender data gap you could read the book by Caroline Criado-Perez, *Invisible women: Exposing data bias in a world designed for men*. Vintage Books.

REFERENCES

Allison, T.R., Symmons, D.P.M., Brammah, T., et al. (2002). Musculoskeletal pain is more generalised among people from ethnic minorities than among white people in Greater Manchester. *Annals of the Rheumatic Diseases*, 61, 151–156.

Biring, S., Burton, A.E., Dunwoody, L., and Kevern, P. (2025). Women's experiences of living with chronic pain: A qualitative meta-synthesis. *British Journal of Health Psychology*, 30, e70023. https://doi.org/10.1111/bjhp.70023.

Brown, V.L., James, A., Hunleth, J., et al. (2024). Believing women: A qualitative exploration of provider disbelief and pain dismissal among women with interstitial cystitis/bladder pain syndrome from the MAPP research network. *International Urogynaecology Journal*, 35(1), 139–148.

Bruce, M., Lopatina, E., Hodge, J., et al. (2023). Understanding the chronic pain journey and coping strategies that patients use to manage their chronic pain: A qualitative patient-led, Canadian study. *BMJ Open*, 13, e072048. doi: 10.1136/bmjopen-2023-072048.

Byrd, W.M. and Clayton, L.A. (2001). Race, medicine, and health care in the United States: A historical survey. *Journal of the National Medical Association*, 93(3 Suppl.), 11S–34S.

Choudhury, Y., Bremner, S.A., Ali, A., et al. (2013). Prevalence and impact of chronic widespread pain in the Bangladeshi and White populations of Tower Hamlets, East London. *Clinical Rheumatology*, 32, 1375–1382.

Clarke, A., Anthony, G., Gray, D., et al. (2012). 'I feel so stupid because I can't give a proper answer …' How older adults describe chronic pain: a qualitative study. *BMC Geriatrics*, 12, 78.

De Ruddere, L., Goubert, L., Prkachin, K.M., et al. (2011). When you dislike patients, pain is taken less seriously. *Pain*, 152(10), 2342–2347.

De Ruddere, L., Goubert, L., Stevens, M., et al. (2013). Discounting pain in the absence of medical evidence is explained by negative evaluation of the patient. *Pain*, 154(5), 669–676.

De Ruddere, L., Goubert, L., Stevens, M.A.L., et al. (2014). Health care professionals' reactions to patient pain: Impact of knowledge about medical evidence and psychosocial influences. *The Journal of Pain*, 15(3), 262–270.

De Ruddere, L. Goubert, L., Vervoort, T., et al. (2012). We discount the pain of others when pain has no medical explanation. *The Journal of Pain*, 13(12), 1198–1205.

Djordjevic, C. (2023). Pain cannot (just) be whatever the person says: A critique of a dogma. *Nursing Philosophy*, 24, e12446. https://doi.org/10.1111/nup.12446.

Drogemuller, A., Du, X., Davis, A., et al. (2025). How do you feel? Physical vocabularies for communicating pain using data physicalization. In M. Karyda, D. Çay, A.K. Bakk, et al. (eds), *Data as experiential knowledge and embodied processes*. https://dl.designresearchsociety.org/eksig/eksig2025/researchpapers/11/.

Evans, S. and De Souza, L. (2008). Dealing with chronic pain: Giving voice to the experiences of mothers with chronic pain and their children. *Qualitative Health Research*, 18(4), 489–500.

Ghoshal, M., Shapiro, H., Todd, K., and Schatman, M.E. (2023). Chronic non-cancer pain management and systemic racism: Time to move toward equal care standards. *Journal of Pain Research*, 2825–2836. https://doi.org/10.2147/JPR.S287314.

Hearn, J., Munday, I., Bullo, S., et al. (2024). Metaphorical markers of pain catastrophising, depression, anxiety, and pain interference in people with chronic pain. *The Journal of Pain*, 26, 104733. https://doi.org/10.1016/j.jpain.2024.104733.

Hoffman, D.E. and Tarzian, A.J. (2001). The girl who cried pain: A bias against women in the treatment of pain. *The Journal of Law, Medicine & Ethics*, 29, 13–27.

Hoffman, K.M., Trawalter, S., Axt, J.R., and Oliver, M.N. (2016). Racial bias in pain assessment and treatment recommendations, and false beliefs about biological differences between blacks and whites. *Proceedings of the National Academy of Sciences (PNAS)*, 113(16), 4296–4301.

Hush, J.M., Refshauge, K., Sullivan, G., et al. (2009). Recovery: What does this mean to patients with low back pain? *Arthritis and Rheumatism*, 61(1), 124–131.

Jarman, A.F., Hwang, A.C., Schleimer, J.P., et al. (2022). Racial disparities in opioid analgesia administration among adult emergency department patients with abdominal pain. *Western Journal of Emergency Medicine*, 23(6), 826–831.

Johnson, N.L., Steffensmeier, K.S., Garvin, L.A., et al. (2024). 'It made me not want to see him …': The role of patient-provider communication in influencing rural-dwelling women veterans' motivation to seek health care for managing chronic pain. *Health Communication*, 39(6), 1161–1174.

Kang, Y., Trewern, L., Jackman, J., et al. (2023). Chronic pain: Definitions and diagnosis. *BMJ*, 381, e076036.

Kenny, D.T., Trevorrow, T., Heard, R., and Faunce, G. (2006). Communicating pain: Do people share an understanding of the meaning of pain descriptors? *Australian Psychologist*, 41(3), 213–218.

Leach, E., Ndosi, M., Jones, G.T., et al. (2024). Access to chronic pain services for adults from minority ethnic groups in the United Kingdom (UK): A scoping review. *Journal of Racial and Ethnic Health Disparities*, 11, 3498–3508.

Lin, J., Drain, A., Goharzad, A., and Mende-Siedlecki, P. (2023). What factors predict anti-Black bias in pain perception? An internal meta-analysis across 40 experimental studies. *Social and Personality Psychology Compass*, e12901. https://doi.org/10.1111/spc3.12901.

Loduca, A., Müller, B.M., Amaral, R., et al. (2014). Chronic pain portrait: Pain perception through the eyes of sufferers. *Revista Dor Sao Paulo*, 15(1), 30–35.

Loftus, S. (2011). Pain and its metaphors: A dialogical approach. *Journal of Medical Humanities*, 31, 213–230.

Maly, A. and Vallerand, A.H. (2018). Neighborhood, socioeconomic, and racial influence on chronic pain. *Pain Management Nursing*, 19(1), 14–22.

McCaffery, M. (1968). *Nursing practice theories related to cognition, bodily pain, and man-environment interactions*. University of Los Angeles.

McCaffery, M. and Robinson, E.S. (2002). Your patient is in pain. Here is how you respond. *Nursing*, 32(1), 36–45

Mende-Siedlecki, P., Qu-Lee, J., Backer, R., and Van Bavel, J.J. (2021). Perceptual contributions to racial bias in pain recognition. *Journal of Experimental Psychology: General*, 148(5), 863–889. https://psycnet.apa.org/doi/10.1037/xge0000600.

Mills, A.M., Shofer, F.S., Boulis, A.K., et al. (2011). Racial disparity in analgesic treatment for ED patients with abdominal or back pain. *American Journal of Emergency Medicine*, 29, 752–756.

Nicholas, M., Vlaeyen, J.W.S., Rief, W., et al. (2019). IASP taskforce for the classification of chronic pain. The IASP classification of chronic pain for ICD-11: chronic primary pain. *Pain*, 160, 28–37.

Oliver, M.N., Wells, K.M., Joy-Gaba, J.A., et al. (2014). Do physicians' implicit views of African Americans affect clinical decision making? *Journal of the American Board of Family Medicine*, 27(2), 177–186.

Paige-Lloyd, E., Lloyd, A., McConnell, A.R., and Hugenberg, K. (2022). Race deficits in pain detection: Medical providers and laypeople fail to accurately perceive pain authenticity among black people. *Social, Psychological and Personality Science*, 13(5), 895–905.

Palmer, B., Macfarlane, G., Afzal, C., et al. (2007). Acculturation and the prevalence of pain amongst South Asian minority ethnic groups in the UK. *Rheumatology*, 46, 1009–1014.

Pasero, C. (2018). Margo McCaffery: Resolute and visionary. *Pain Management Nursing*, 19(2), 89–91.

Patrick-Smith, M. and Bull, S. (2024). Medical student perceptions of gender and pain: A systematic review of the literature. *BMC Medicine*, 22, 434. https://doi.org/10.1186/s12916-024-03660-0.

Reibel, M.D. and Pearson, D. (2017). Beyond the pain: A look into the experiences of women living with fibromyalgia. *International Journal of Human Caring*, 21(2), 68–76.

Rice, K., Connoy, L., and Webster, F. (2024). Gendered worlds of pain: Women, marginalization and chronic pain. *The Journal of Pain*, 11, 104626.

Scarry, E. (1985). *The body in pain: The making and unmaking of the world*. Oxford University Press.

Schubiner, H., Jackson, B., Molina, K.M., et al. (2023). Racism as a source of pain. *Journal of General Internal Medicine*, 38(7), 1729–1734.

Shakespeare, T. (2021). 'This is going to hurt me more than it hurts you': The problem of pain. In P. Wemyss-Gorman (ed.), *Innovative approaches to chronic pain: Understanding the experience of pain and suffering and the role of healing*. Jessica Kingsley Publishers.

Strand, N.H., Mariano, E.R., Goree, J.H., et al. (2021). Racism in pain medicine: We can and should do more. *Mayo Clinical Proceedings*, 96(6), 1394–1400.

Wuytack, F. and Miller, P. (2011). The lived experience of fibromyalgia in female patients: A phenomenological study. *Chiropractic & Manual Therapies*, 19(1), 22. https://doi.org/10.1186/2045-709x-19-22.

Yorkston, K.M., Johnson, K., Boesflug, E., et al. (2010). Communicating about the experience of pain and fatigue in disability. *Quality of Life Research*, 19(2), 243–251.

4

WHY IS IT SO HARD TO MANAGE YOUR OWN PAIN?

INTRODUCTION

This chapter explores the challenges of managing persistent pain. Pain medication only helps some patients and, even for those, they are then often faced with managing side effects of the long-term use of medicine (Gauntlett-Gilbert & Brook, 2018). Thinking about how to cope with living with persistent pain can feel overwhelming and many people go to pain management services hoping to have their pain removed or at least controlled. After all, this is how we approach most of our other ailments; we take them to the health professional and ask to be made better. This kind of approach works for acute (short-term) pain, but 'falls short for most chronic pain' (Glare et al., 2025, p. 202).

In 2004 the International Association for the Study of Pain and the European Federation of IASP Chapters (EFIC) issued a joint declaration which stated that the treatment of pain should be a human right (Lipman, 2005). In 2010 this formed the 'Declaration of Montreal' (shared on the IASP website, which is listed in the resources at the end of this chapter) where three key points were made:

1. The right of all people to have access to pain management without discrimination.

DOI: 10.4324/9781003649854-4

2. The right of people in pain to acknowledgment of their pain and to be informed about how it can be assessed and managed.
3. The right of all people with pain to have access to appropriate assessment and treatment of the pain by adequately trained health care professionals.

(IASP, n.d.)

However, as the numbers of people living with persistent pain continue to rise, our National Health Service here in the United Kingdom, where I am based, increasingly struggles to cope. This is not a surprise, for its original function was to address acute, not chronic care. The Darzi (2024) report lays bare the problems facing the NHS, which range from difficulty accessing GPs to long waiting lists. Furthermore, research from Healthwatch England (2021) quoted in the Darzi report, highlighted that 82 per cent of people on lists, received no help at all with pain relief, physiotherapy or mental health support while waiting. Connelly (2020) estimated wait times ranged from six weeks to two years for pain management programmes.

The impact of a long wait is serious and not unique to the United Kingdom. For example, Liddy and colleagues (2024) explored the wait times and the impact of living with chronic pain via a waiting-room survey in chronic pain clinics held in Canada. Patients were asked how long they had waited for their appointment since being referred, to rate their quality of life, as well as to indicate which (if any) health professionals they had seen while waiting. Around 25 per cent of the 593 participants had waited 6 months to 1 year for their appointment, and around 20 per cent reported waiting over 1 year. For example, one participant wrote: 'I had to call repeatedly to ensure that progress was being made. I finally received an appointment for June 2022. Had I not repeatedly followed up I would still be waiting while dealing with unmanaged chronic pain' (Liddy et al., 2024, p. 7). Participants also wrote about difficulties navigating the health system, problems with (lost) referrals, decreased quality of life, and the distress they experienced while waiting. The distress this causes is clearly outlined in the following quote:

> I called many times over the summer and fall to get different answers. I wasn't told the real truth of the wait time until the fall. I was then told it would still be 18 months probably! This is disgusting. Specialists and people who are answering the calls should be honest!! Stop giving people in pain HOPE, when that HOPE will not be coming for years!
>
> (Liddy et al., 2024, p. 7)

Long waiting times for accessing pain management support are problematic. After all, the sooner a person has access to pain management programmes, the sooner they learn skills that will help them to cope with their persistent pain better. It is important to note here that, although pain management programmes typically focus on the person living with pain, it is very difficult to manage persistent pain by yourself. Whilst there are, of course, things the person living with pain can do for themselves, there are also things that friends, carers, health professionals, employers, and national leaders can (and must do), to better help people to live well in spite of their pain.

When a person lives with persistent pain, they might rely on behaviours that were helpful in the past when they experienced acute pain. These might include resting (not moving) an affected arm or leg. This is often good practice when you live with acute pain because resting protects the limb from further injury. But not moving a limb that is affected by persistent pain can store up longer-term problems. Often the protection behaviour learned from acute pain experiences makes the situation worse. Glare and colleagues (2025, p. 202) explain how '[i]nactivity can result in physical deconditioning, stiffness and weight gain', all of which can increase the persistent pain. Worse still, as people lose confidence in their ability to cope with their pain, they can become overwhelmed with the worries they have about their pain getting even worse in the future. Being stuck in your own worries impacts on your wellbeing and on your relationships, and it can increase the stress experienced by yourself and those loved ones around you. Glare and colleagues (2025) suggest that rather than cure from pain, the goal of treatment for those living with persistent pain should be focused on improving function in spite of the pain. This, I think, is at the heart of why managing persistent pain is so difficult. We are taught from a young age that if something hurts, we should rest it. The opposite is often true when living with persistent pain. Self-management of persistent pain is therefore challenging on a number of fronts.

BUT WHAT DO WE MEAN BY SELF-MANAGEMENT OF PERSISTENT PAIN?

Self-management of persistent pain has been defined as a person's ability to manage their symptoms and their treatment as well as the physical and psychological impact of living with persistent pain. It is also about the person making the lifestyle changes that are needed in order to live with persistent pain (Karadag et al., 2025). It relies on people moving from being passive receivers of treatments from health professionals, to being actively involved in their own care (Jonkman et al., 2016).

It will not have escaped your notice that the phrase 'self-management' puts the responsibility for managing the pain on the 'self'. In other words, the focus is on the person who is living with persistent pain. No attention is paid to the

> [...] context or background of the person's life, their support network (or lack thereof), their health literacy (or lack thereof), their financial capacity (or lack thereof), their social capital (or lack thereof) and their relationship with their health professionals (or lack thereof). And yet, the person living with pain is expected to cope.
>
> (Rodham, 2020, p. 53)

Indeed, given so much of our life context impacts on our ability to manage, it seems unfair to expect people to self-manage. Living well with a pain condition is not something that can be done without support from health professionals. Likewise, how can health professionals offer advice or instructions unless they have some understanding of the context in which their patient lives. Surely the health professional needs to know about their patient's life context to ensure that recommendations and instructions will work in that context?

Interestingly, the original approach to pain management was 'supported self-management'. For example, Cameron and Stewart (2012, p. 231), writing in Scotland about persistent pain management, noted that the increase in numbers of people living with long-term conditions had 'driven government policy to advocate the promotion of patient responsibility for the day-to-day management of their own condition, and the positive role health care professionals can, and should, play to support patients'. What the supported element might look like, though, at that time was unclear, which meant it was also unclear as to whether health professionals should act as a source of guidance and advice, or perhaps collaborate with the patients to find the best patient-centred way forward? Should health professionals actively teach strategies? How long should the support last? How sustainable was ongoing support in times of shortage of funds, services, and so forth? Amidst this uncertainty, somewhere along the line, the 'supported' element has disappeared. The shift from 'supported self-management' to simply 'self-management' may well be in response to the increasing numbers of people living with long-term conditions. The health service in the United Kingdom, as I have already noted, is struggling to cope. It is therefore not surprising that opportunities to streamline services will be taken. People who are lucky enough to make it to the top of the long waiting lists can then access a pain management programme and are discharged with the intention that they self-manage. However, the dropping of the word 'supported' from 'self-management', the lack of agreement about what self-management is, and the failure to fully explore a patient's life context leaves room for negative judgement of those people who do not successfully self-manage.

In trying to understand what positive self-management might look like, Van de Velde and colleagues (2019, p. 10) focused on reviewing chronic conditions (not just persistent pain) and highlighted that responsibility for managing remains firmly on the shoulders of the individual:

> Self-management is the intrinsically controlled ability of an active, responsible, informed and autonomous individual to live with the medical, role and emotional consequences of his chronic condition(s) in partnership with his social network and the healthcare provider(s).

I found their paper really interesting because, through reviewing already published papers that focused on self-management of chronic conditions, they were able to identify the ingredients that are needed for successful self-management. They did what is called a 'concept analysis' to try to make sense of all the different elements that the journal articles they reviewed had reported as contributing to successful self-management. Their concept analysis resulted in the identification of ten attributes, which I have listed in Table 4.1.

Table 4.1 *Ten attributes identified by Van de Velde and colleagues (2019) for self-managing chronic conditions*

Attributes	*Expectations*
Attribute 1	The person must actively take part in the care process
Attribute 2	The person must take responsibility for the care process
Attribute 3	The person must have a positive way of coping with difficulty
Attribute 4	The person must be informed about the condition, disease, and treatment
Attribute 5	The person must express their needs, values, and priorities
Attribute 6	The person must be open to a reciprocal relationship with health professionals
Attribute 7	The person must be open to social support
Attribute 8	The person must recognise that self-management is a lifetime task
Attribute 9	The person must have the following skills: Problem solving, decision-making, using resources, forming a patient-health care provider partnership, proactive action planning
Attribute 10	The person must be able to manage medical, role, and emotional aspects

In the next section of this chapter, the list of attributes developed by Van de Velde and colleagues (2019) are used as a framework to show why managing your own pain is so difficult.

ATTRIBUTE 1: THE PERSON MUST ACTIVELY TAKE PART IN THE CARE PROCESS

This attribute suggests that the person who lives with pain must play their part and become actively involved in their treatment planning and the management of their condition. As I have pointed out in previous chapters, people who live with pain are often faced with an uphill battle of convincing health professionals that their pain is both real and difficult to live with. It is really hard to measure something that is both invisible and a personal experience, not least because it is very hard to explain pain to another person. This attribute is therefore difficult to achieve because of the in-built power imbalance in the health system. Traditionally health professionals are thought of as experts who tell those who are unwell what to do. This traditional expectation is difficult to shake off. The work of Dupont and colleagues (2025) shows that GPs make assumptions about their patients' needs which do not always match what the patients in the research said they needed. When there is a mismatch in assumptions combined with a power imbalance, it can be hard for the person in pain to play an active part. After all, people can only play an active part if they are respected, believed, and listened to. In my opinion, this attribute is a little one-sided. I think health professionals should play their part too, and should recognise that the patient is an expert in their pain and their experience.

ATTRIBUTE 2: THE PERSON MUST TAKE RESPONSIBILITY FOR THE CARE PROCESS

Having established in Attribute 1 that a patient should play an active role in the care process, this attribute states that they must also take responsibility 'for the care regardless whether or not there is a social network of family, friends and other proxies on whom the patient can rely or can consult with trust' (Van de Velde et al., 2019, p. 4). The core focus of this attribute is taking responsibility for day-to-day care. This is a very big ask, for it is made clear that this is an expectation that is held regardless of each person's life context. Someone who has a supportive and loving family, who is informed about and understands their pain condition, who understands the treatment and therapy options that are available to them, and who is able to express themselves assertively may be able to take responsibility for the care process, but the ability to do so does not lie wholly in their control. They are reliant on the health professionals allowing them to do so.

ATTRIBUTE 3: THE PERSON MUST HAVE A POSITIVE WAY OF COPING WITH DIFFICULTY

Coping with persistent pain is not easy. Attribute 3 requires people who live with chronic conditions to have a positive way of coping with difficulty. Recognition is given to the fact that people who live with chronic conditions inevitably experience anger and frustration. The ability to cope positively with these difficult emotions is said to be a key part of the process of learning to self-manage. In effect what is focused on here is the ability to cope when facing difficult situations. This requires a person to have reached a level of acceptance about what has happened to them.

A key aspect of positive coping when a person lives with persistent pain is to learn how to pace. Some people call this 'Spoon Theory'. Spoon Theory was developed by Christine Miserandino (2003) as a way of explaining how she coped with the impact of living with lupus. Miserandino wanted to find a way to explain to her friend how lupus impacted on her daily life. She and her friend were in a restaurant and so Miserandino used spoons as a way of representing her energy for the day. There were twelve spoons. She explained that something that seems as simple as getting up and going to work involves many decisions about where to spend your limited amount of energy. Before you can get dressed, you need to take your medicine. You have to take your medicine with food, so you need to make breakfast. Then you need to shower. That is potentially three spoons used up before you have even left the house. Miserandino's friend soon began to realise how difficult it is to organise your day when you have limited energy. Spoon Theory has become a really clear way of explaining something known as 'pacing'. Pacing is a key part of learning to live with long-term conditions such as persistent pain. It is a difficult skill to master, not least because our days do not divide up into neat packages and we often find it hard to come to terms with being unable to do everything we used to do. If we do not learn to pace, we can overdo things on one day and then suffer the next with a flare-up of our pain (this is often called the 'boom-and-bust' cycle). It can be hard to see that slowing things down and taking more rests than maybe we want to can, in the longer term, help reduce the flare-ups of our pain, and so allow us to do more.

ATTRIBUTE 4: THE PERSON MUST BE INFORMED ABOUT THE CONDITION, DISEASE, AND TREATMENT

This attribute puts the onus on the person with pain to obtain and develop their knowledge about their condition and treatment. In some ways this is a reasonable expectation: After all, if you are to cope with persistent pain, you need to understand your pain condition. However, the health professional ought to play an active role here too. They should explain the condition to their patients in ways that the patients can understand, and they should also check that their patients have understood. A key barrier, though, is the literacy level of the population. In the United Kingdom, for example, the average reading age is around 11 years old (Department for Education, 2024). People with low literacy levels may struggle to find trustworthy information in an accessible format. Self-management programmes ought to cater to this level, instead of asserting that it is the responsibility of the person with pain.

Therefore, whilst I agree that it is important that people try to understand their conditions, I also think that it is the responsibility of the health professionals both to share information in an accessible way and to check that their patients have understood their condition and the treatment options.

ATTRIBUTE 5: THE PERSON MUST EXPRESS THEIR NEEDS, VALUES, AND PRIORITIES

This attribute recognises that successful self-management should be based on the patient's 'perceived problems and their personal perceptions of their condition in the context in which they live' (Van de Velde et al., 2019, p. 6). Whilst it is great to see life context being recognised, there is possibly a hint of judgement in the decision to use the words 'perceived problems' and 'perceptions of their condition'. Surely, if a person identifies a problem, then it should be seen as a problem, not as a 'perceived' problem. Similarly, surely the person's perceptions about their condition are what is important? In the pain context, this goes back to the McCaffery statement about pain being whatever the person experiencing that pain says it is. That said, a more generous reading of the wording is that self-management should be based on how the person sees the world (their problems and their condition). This reading of the attribute is more positive.

However, the statement that the person must express their needs assumes that a person will be able to do so. I've already mentioned the impact of literacy levels on people's ability to understand information. This also impacts on people's ability to express themselves. And telling someone else what your needs, values, and priorities are is not an easy thing to do. Even if you have the ability to express yourself, you may be concerned about how your needs, values, and priorities may be judged. It seems to me that this is an attribute that, at face value, is reasonable and important, but one that on closer examination is more complex, putting the onus on the person in pain and potentially ignoring the role of the health professional.

ATTRIBUTE 6: THE PERSON MUST BE OPEN TO A RECIPROCAL RELATIONSHIP WITH HEALTH PROFESSIONALS

The word reciprocal is embedded in this attribute. Reciprocal means 'two-way'. I wonder why it was not phrased in the following way: 'The person and the health professional(s) must be open to a reciprocal relationship'. As it is currently phrased, it is as if the person with the chronic condition is in need of reminding that there should be a reciprocal relationship, not the health professional. The slight tweak I have suggested makes it explicit that this is to be a collaboration. Given the challenges I have outlined in previous chapters, where I have shared the experiences of people who live with persistent pain and who describe being belittled, not listened to, not believed, I imagine that being told that they must be open to a reciprocal relationship will possibly not be well received. Nevertheless, this attribute does focus on shared expertise. This sounds good. It sounds collaborative. It sounds almost like a partnership. But, Van de Velde and colleagues (2019, p. 6) say that:

> The person is open to receiving feedback from the healthcare provider, making it possible to continue the care process. When patients are self-managing, it implies that they are in favour of collaboration and guidance of physicians and other healthcare providers. This means that a patient-provider partnership has to be built, in which the patient and the provider occupy equal positions and co-operatively work together. This also means that the patient needs to know when to report changes to healthcare providers.

The framing of this is that the aim is for collaboration – the phrase 'equal positions' is used, but my reading of this is that it is more about the patient cooperating. It is the patient who needs to be open to feedback from the provider. If the relationship was truly reciprocal, the health professional would also be open to feedback. Later in same paragraph that the quote is taken from, it is suggested that patients be 'assertive' in order to allow appropriate interaction with the health professional. So once again, the work falls to the patient, who has to be assertive in order to interact. The patient has to be open to feedback and, if they want to offer feedback, they have to learn to be assertive in order to be heard. This does not sound reciprocal.

ATTRIBUTE 7: THE PERSON MUST BE OPEN TO SOCIAL SUPPORT

I completely agree with the essence of this attribute. Indeed, the literature shows that support is essential (see Cordero, 2024; De Matos & Bernardes, 2023). However, I am bothered by the wording – that a person must be open to social support. Some people have very little support. Perhaps they have no family. Perhaps they have family who are not supportive. Either way, they lack support. What does being open to social support look like? What kind of social support should they be open to? And who decides? If a person with minimal social support was referred to a support group, would they be required to attend? I can think of people with whom I have worked who would prefer not to talk in a group setting. This is not something these people would have been open to doing. And why should they be, for such groups are not for everyone. Yet the phrasing here suggests that they would have to be open to doing so.

On the other hand, we know from the research evidence that family and community support is an important element of pain self-management. Indeed, there is evidence that social support helps people to reframe their pain, reduces pain-related thoughts, and even lowers the perceived intensity of pain (Weiß et al., 2024). So it is important that those who lack social support should be helped to access it. In order to do this well, a person-centred approach will need to be taken to ensure that the right kind of support is put in place. Not everyone will want practical or emotional support, so if someone politely turns down an offer of support because it is not needed, does that make them open or closed to support? How will the polite refusal be viewed. Will the person be labelled as 'not engaging'? The key way to establish what the right kind of social support is will be to take the time to understand the person's life context. For example, rather than referring a person to a support group, it might be more appropriate to help the person to learn to ask for the support they need. With this in mind, I remember working with many people who had family and friends desperate to offer support, yet the person coming to terms with living with pain was reluctant to ask for help for fear of becoming a burden to their loved ones. For example, I interviewed 'Stella' (Rodham, 2015, p. 84) who spoke of her concern for her family. She did not want them to worry about her, and she did not want to become a burden, so she worked hard to put up a front:

> And people don't want you being always miserable in front of them. My husband had enough to cope with me having it, let alone being sort of down you know. Certainly not depressed, but a bit, when you are in pain and your life is a bit restricted, you are not going to go around with a great beaming smile are you?

ATTRIBUTE 8: THE PERSON MUST RECOGNISE THAT SELF-MANAGEMENT IS A LIFETIME TASK

This attribute requires the person living with persistent pain to have reached a level of acceptance that their condition is life changing and is likely something they will need to manage for the rest of their lives. The impact of persistent pain touches all parts of a person's life and so requires multiple changes and adaptations. The Health Talk Online website mentions that many of the people that they talked to felt that coming to terms with and understanding that their pain was likely to be a permanent part of their life was vital for them to be able to learn to live their life in spite of their chronic pain. The participants spoke of how the alternative to acceptance was 'pointless anger, aggression and bitterness that could ruin the person's life and destroy their most important relationships'. In short, this attribute is not an easy item to tick off on a 'to do' list. It is something which takes time to come to terms with. A researcher called Cathy Charmaz (1983) wrote about the journey to acceptance involving grieving for your imagined futures. Similarly, Gunning and Taladay-Carter (2023) note that when an individual experiences the onset of illness, they must grieve their physical abilities, their identity, and their dreams lost because of their illness. Many of the things an individual may have planned for their future may now need to be rethought at the same time as they adjust to the physical and emotional (and financial and social, etc.) impacts. There is no doubt that this is an important attribute, but I think it is worth highlighting that it is a challenging process and is one that could be achieved with support from the health profession.

ATTRIBUTE 9: THE PERSON MUST HAVE A RANGE OF SKILLS

These skills are largely a summary of the attributes 1 through to 8 and require patients to be proactive in their approach to managing their pain. Patients will need to have the ability to learn to be flexible, to problem-solve as new challenges arise, and to make informed decisions that will help rather than hinder their how they manage their pain and set their own goals. They will need to be able to access (and hence to know how and where to access) resources that will help with their pain management. In this attribute, the skill of forming a patient-provider partnership is once again mentioned. And once again, the onus here is on the patient to develop the partnership. This attribute alone sounds exhausting to read in its entirely in the journal article.

ATTRIBUTE 10: THE PERSON MUST BE ABLE TO MANAGE MEDICAL, ROLE, AND EMOTIONAL ASPECTS

This attribute focuses on three layers of self-management, as follows.

In terms of **medical management**: This focuses on condition-specific tasks, such as taking medication appropriately, managing symptoms, and reducing lifestyle risk factors, perhaps through regular exercise, healthy eating, and/or stopping smoking.

In terms of **role management**: This is about patients maintaining, changing, or creating new meaningful behaviours or life roles that enable them to live well with their condition. This also involves the more practical skill of pacing in order to cope with the fatigue and reduced mobility that can come with living with persistent pain.

In terms of **emotional management**: This is about the person's ability to cope with and manage their emotions. Failure to do this has an impact on a person's ability to self-manage.

ATTRIBUTE SUMMARY

Having explored the ten attributes for successful self-management that Van der Velde and colleagues (2019) listed, I feel exhausted. There are a lot of expectations placed upon people living with persistent pain if they are expected to develop all ten attributes. There is little doubt that each attribute in this list (possibly with small tweaks to some of the wording) is important and it is difficult to argue with the need for them. However, little attention is paid to the emotional experience of living with long-term conditions, other than the attribute that states that people with chronic conditions must have a positive way of dealing with difficulty. This is an important omission and one that Boersma and Flink (2025, p. 1) highlighted when they said that the 'emotional component of pain is easily forgotten in the popular, scientific and clinical contexts'. They also draw attention to how the chronic pain experience is impacted by relationships and social experiences. They write of how people with persistent pain experience stigma, disbelief, social exclusion, and so on. All these things will impact on a person's ability to develop these ten attributes. Furthermore, there is little attention paid to the role of the health professional. The person with the chronic condition has been looked at in splendid isolation. The need for a collaborative approach is in the main, not mentioned (aside from Attribute 6, which insists the person should be open to a reciprocal relationship). It seems to me that we are expecting a lot from people who are learning to cope with the impact of their condition on all aspects of their life. The focus of these ten attributes is on the person who has the chronic condition. We must remember that we each live in our own life context and how we live will impact on our ability to develop these attributes. We also need to remember that, as with everything, everything changes and, as we age, so too will the way in which we experience our persistent pain. Self-management is therefore something that is also ever changing in order to adapt to the changes in our lives.

SO WHY IS IT SO HARD TO MANAGE YOUR OWN PAIN?

It is interesting that the attributes that were developed based on the papers included in the review by Van de Velde and colleagues (2019) focus attention on what the person with the chronic condition can do. This is a one-sided perspective about self-management. In a previous book, I wrote about pain self-management and highlighted how there had been a shift away from supported self-management towards self-management with all the emphasis on what the person with pain could do to cope (Rodham, 2020). I labelled this the 'blame, shame, and inflame game' because I believe that no one can manage, let alone live well with, a chronic health condition such as persistent pain all by themselves. If someone is living with a long-term condition, of course they have a responsibility to do what they can for themselves, but they will need ongoing help and support from the health profession too. Van de Velde and colleagues (2019) also recognise that achieving what they call 'optimal' self-management behaviour is difficult and needs a lot of effort from the person with pain. They highlight that it is crucial that health professionals 'recognise the current level and readiness for self-management of the individual client'. I would go further than this and say that recognising the level is not enough – understanding the things that impact on a person's readiness is more helpful. In short, it is really hard for a person to manage their own pain because such a lot is expected of that person. The person in pain has to find a way to be heard and then to be believed. In order to be believed they may have to overcome a number of biases (e.g., those based on race, gender, socioeconomic status). They are expected to maintain a positive approach to coping and to take responsibility for communicating with their health professionals. In order to be listened to, the work of De Ruddere and colleagues (2011) has shown that they also need to be likeable. They need to do as they are told by the health profession, yet they are also expected to play an active role in the care process. All of this while coming to terms with a long-term condition, keeping their life running as best they can, and learning to live well in spite of their persistent pain.

FURTHER RESOURCES

Declaration of Montreal (2010). Available at https://www.iasp-pain.org/advocacy/iasp-statements/access-to-pain-management-declaration-of-montreal/ [accessed 31 January 2026].

Health Talk Online: Chronic pain. https://healthtalk.org/experiences/chronic-pain/coming-terms-chronic-pain/ [accessed 17 January 2026].

NHS (2023). *Health Literacy Toolkit*, 2nd edition. NHS England.

REFERENCES

Boersma, K. and Flink, I.K. (2025). Key aspects concerning the role of emotion in the chronic pain experience. *Current Opinion in Psychology*, 62, 102000. https://doi.org/10.1016/j.copsyc.2025.102000.

Cameron, P.A. and Stewart, C. (2012). The need to define chronic pain self-management. *Journal of Pain Management*, 5(3), 231–236.

Charmaz, K. (1983). Loss of self: A fundamental form of suffering in the chronically ill. *Sociology of Health and Illness*, 5(2), 168–195.

Connelly, D. (2020). Some patients with chronic pain face waiting years to see a specialist. *Pharmaceutical Journal*. doi.10.1211/PJ.2020.20207637.

Cordero, D. (2024). The healing others: The essential role of social support on chronic pain management. *Korean Journal of Pain*, 37(3), 280–282.

Darzi, A. (2024). *Independent investigation of the National Health Service in England*. Department of Health and Social Care, UK. Available at https://www.gov.uk/government/publications/independent-investigation-of-the-nhs-in-england [accessed 31 January 2026].

De Matos, M.O. and Bernardes, S.F. (2023). Helpful social support for chronic pain in long-term care residents: 'With a little help I manage on my own'. *Nursing Open*, 10, 6326–6335. https://doi.org/10.1002/nop2.1881.

De Ruddere, L., Goubert, L., Prkachin, K.M., et al. (2011). When you dislike patients, pain is taken less seriously. *Pain*, 152(10), 2342–2347.

Department for Education (2024). *Survey of adult skills 2023 (PIAAC): National Report for England research report*. Department for Education, UK.

Dupont, D., Brinkmöller, S., Carter, S., et al. (2025). Exploring physician and patient perspectives on expectations and role models towards chronic pain treatment in general practice: A qualitative cross-sectional study. *Healthcare*, 13, 187. https://doi.org/10.3390/healthcare13020187.

Gauntlett-Gilbert, J. and Brook, P. (2018). Living well with chronic pain: The role of pain management programmes. *BJE Education*, 18(1), 3–7.

Glare, P., Mahendran, M., and Weiss, A.D. (2025). Update on chronic pain management. *Internal Medicine Journal*, 55, 200–206.

Gunning, J.N. and Taladay-Carter, C. (2023). Grieving 'The death of possibility': Memorable messages of (dis)enfranchised loss in invisible physical illness. *Health Communication*, 39(10), 2152–2162. https://doi.org/10.1080/10410236.2023.2257942.

Healthwatch England (2021). What are people telling us about delays to hospital care and treatment? https://nds.healthwatch.co.uk/sites/default/files/reports_library/20211108%2520Healthwatch%2520England%2520Elective%2520Care%2520Briefing.pdf [accessed 7 February 2026].

IASP, International Association for the Study of Pain (n.d.) https://www.iasp-pain.org/advocacy/iasp-statements/access-to-pain-management-declaration-of-montreal/.

Jonkman, N.H., Schuurmans, M.J., Jaarsma, T., et al. (2016). Self-management interventions: Proposal and validation of a new operational definition. *Journal of Clinical Epidemiology*, 80, 34–42. doi: 10.1016/j.jclinepi.2016.08.001

Karadag, P., Taylor, J., and Burton, A. (2025). Self-management and coping in young adults with chronic pain: A reflexive thematic analysis. *Journal of Health Psychology*. doi: 10.1177/13591053251344236.

Liddy, C., Cooper, L., Bellingham, G., et al. (2024). Patient-reported wait times and the impact of living with chronic pain on their quality of life: A waiting room survey in chronic pain clinics in Ontario, Manitoba and Quebec. *Canadian Journal of Pain*, 8(1), 2345612. https://doi.org/10.1080/24740527.2024.2345612.

Lipman, A.G. (2005). Pain as a human right: The 2004 Global Day Against Pain. *Journal of Pain & Palliative Care Pharmacotherapy*, 19(3), 85–100.

Miserandino, C. (2003). *The Spoon Theory*, reproduced for the Lymphoma Action Conference, 2020. Available at https://lymphoma-action.org.uk/sites/default/files/media/documents/2020-05/Spoon%20theory%20by%20Christine%20Miserandino.pdf [accessed 31 January 2026].

Rodham, K. (2015). *Learning to cope with CRPS/RSD: Putting life first and pain second*. Singing Dragon.

Rodham, K. (2020). *Self-management for persistent pain: The blame, shame and inflame game?* Palgrave Macmillan.

Van de Velde, D., De Zutter, F., Satink, T., et al. (2019). Delineating the concept of self-management in chronic conditions: A concept analysis. *BMJ Open*, 9, e027775. doi:10.1136/bmjopen-2018-027775.

Weiß, M., Jachnik, A., Lampe, E.C., et al. (2024). Differential effects of everyday-life social support on chronic pain. *BMC Neurology*, 24, 301. doi: 10.1186/s12883-024-03792-z.

5

IS IT TRUE THAT LAUGHTER AND SWEARING CAN HELP WITH PAIN?

INTRODUCTION

Researchers have explored whether swearing and laughter (though not necessarily at the same time) can reduce pain. This research generates lots of headlines. For example: 'Laughter really is the best medicine', 'Laugh away the pain', 'Laughter is a natural painkiller', and 'Swearing is a really powerful painkiller'. In this chapter, I look at the research behind the headlines and share what is currently known about swearing and laughter, and their potential to reduce pain.

Humour and swearing are tricky places to tread. They are very personal yet can easily cause offence. What one person considers to be a swear word, another uses as punctuation. What one person finds funny leaves another person cold. Nevertheless, there is a growing body of research on each of these topics that might be relevant for people who are living with persistent pain. I will do my best to give a clear overview of these topics, while trying to avoid causing you, the reader, any offence. I will share what I have learned from the research evidence about how laughter and swearing can impact on our wellbeing, before exploring whether laughter and swearing might benefit people living with persistent pain.

DOI: 10.4324/9781003649854-5

LAUGHTER

Laughter is known to have many beneficial effects. It reduces stress, improves our mood, and it can also improve our communication and our social relationships (Spytska, 2024). Laughing is said to be good for us, indeed, in the United Kingdom, 'laughter is the best medicine' is a well-known phrase. According to Bennett and Lengacher (2006), laughter is how we communicate our response to a humorous experience. But what counts as humour can be difficult to define. There are perhaps things that you find extremely funny, but others among your family or friends do not. By way of example, I can remember 20-plus years ago watching a video of an experiment where a teacher stood at the front of their classroom and just started laughing. Pretty soon, a few students started to giggle and, not long after that, the whole class was laughing and that person's lesson got off to a positive start. I thought I'd give it a go the next time I had a huge class (almost 200 students) to teach. My laughter attempt, though, fell completely flat. I think I was too self-conscious and perhaps should have kept laughing a little longer in the face of the students bemused silence. Once I stopped and explained what I was trying to do (to see if laughter would be infectious), the students chose that moment to fall about laughing. So I suppose I succeeded in an indirect way. My students did not find my laughing humorous, but they found my epic fail hilarious.

This is one of the things that makes this topic complex – different things make us laugh. So even though we know that humour can bring a variety of physiological, psychological, and social benefits, Warren and colleagues (2021, p. 41) note that 'Neither the Three Stooges, nor cat memes will help someone overcome personal or social hurdles if the person does not think that stooges or grumpy cats are funny'. Furthermore, they highlighted that people and organisations who try but fail to be funny tend to be viewed negatively. So it seems I had a forgiving group of students the day I tried to make them laugh. This means that understanding what it is that makes something funny is really important. Apparently, there are more than

20 theories that try to explain what makes something funny, but there is, as yet, no agreement about what it actually is that makes something funny (Warren et al., 2021).

Nevertheless, there are a growing number of researchers who are investigating the role(s) that humour plays in our lives (Basler et al., 2025). Indeed, there are academic journals dedicated to this research (see, for example, *The European Journal of Humour Research*). There is also an International Society of Humour Studies which publishes its own journal simply called *Humor*. There is even a word for someone who studies laughter: gelotologist. In terms of using laughter in therapy, the idea is to use of humour and playful activities to promote health and wellbeing (Kim and Choi, 2025). Approaches include laughter yoga and clown therapy.

Laughter yoga

Dr Madan Kataria is said to have invented laughter yoga. You can search for his name on YouTube and find many videos of him sharing his laughter yoga. I find it very difficult to feel grumpy when I watch one of his videos. He is clear that you can just start laughing, you do not need to start with a genuine laugh: the point is that you just laugh and keep on laughing. Invariably, this turns into a real laugh. For Dr Kataria, it is the act of laughing that is important.

Laughter yoga is a practice that combines laughter exercises with yogic breathing techniques. The aim is to increase a person's physical and mental wellbeing by harnessing the physiological and psychological benefits of laughter (Sharma et al., 2024). The laughter triggers endorphins. Endorphins are natural pain-relieving and mood-enhancing chemicals in our brains. The breathing exercises activate our body's relaxation system, which reduces our stress hormones and helps us to feel calm. Combining both the laughter and the breathing techniques is said to enhance our feelings of wellbeing.

We often think about laughter and laughing as taking place with other people. However, Gonot-Schoupinsky and Garip (2019) drew from the principles of laughter yoga and designed something they called the 'Laughie' to be used for what they termed 'solo laughing'. They gathered together a group of participants who were invited to make their own Laughie. A Laughie is a recording you make of yourself laughing unprompted for one minute. Participants were told that for the next seven days they had to listen to their Laughie and, at the same time, laugh with it (once in the morning, once in the afternoon, and once in the evening). Most participants responded positively to the experience. For example, a Laughie participant said: 'Sometimes I was laughing so much and I was like oh my God, what, it's just funny just to hear my laughter' (Gonot-Schoupinsky & Garip, 2019, p. 60). Their participants reported increased wellbeing and the Laughie was considered to be enjoyable and convenient to use. This suggests the Laughie may be a feasible and easy-to-use intervention for improving wellbeing in healthy adults. So it is clear that laughing and laughter have a positive impact on our wellbeing, but what about their impact on pain? Can laughter and laughing help people who live with persistent pain?

Laughter and pain

A research team in Texas, in the United States, wanted to explore whether laughing in response to something funny would bring relief from pain. Lapierre and colleagues (2019) set out to investigate whether what they called 'mirthful laughter' might influence pain tolerance. I was excited when I read the first line of the summary of this study because it mentioned chronic pain. Hurrah, I thought, someone has completed a study with people who are living with persistent pain.

However, as I read on, I quickly realised that the participants in this study were healthy American students. The research team made the students do something called eccentric resistance exercise. This is a form of strength training that makes a person's muscles sore a few days after the exercise. It was this muscle soreness that was used to simulate the experience of chronic pain. Participants came to the laboratory three times over the course of a week for each leg. Visit 1 induced muscle soreness in one leg. Visit 2 tested muscle soreness and pain tolerance and involved watching a video. Visit 3 involved testing muscle soreness and pain tolerance. This was repeated the following week for the other leg. On the first visit, participants were randomised so that some watched a comedy video in the first week and an uninteresting documentary in the second week, whilst others watched the uninteresting documentary first. For the comedy video, participants were invited to pick a video of a stand-up comedian of their choice. This ensured that their particular humour preference was met. The uninteresting documentary was chosen by the investigators. Arguably what is deemed interesting is as unique as what is deemed humorous. For example, I recently took a friend to visit the nearby Brickworks Museum. I had been curious see what would be included in such a place. My friend, Rebecca, reluctantly came along (because she is a good friend). At the end of our visit, she admitted she had found it quite interesting. So what at face value was perceived as uninteresting, ended up being a place where we spent a happy couple of hours. I wonder if the same might be said for the 'uninteresting' documentaries. I digress. The researchers reported that 30 minutes of watching a comedy that made participants laugh positively influenced their pain tolerance compared to their tolerance when watching the uninteresting documentary. So comedy did provide relief from pain. But, as the researchers themselves noted, their study needs to be repeated with people who are actually living with chronic pain and not experiencing temporary muscle ache.

Humour training

Researchers in Hong Kong designed a humour therapy programme for 36 older adults who lived with persistent pain in a residential care home (Tse et al., 2010). The programme was delivered over the course of one-hour sessions (once a week for eight weeks). Each participant was given a blank portfolio called 'My happy collection' that they were encouraged to fill with examples of funny photos, jokes, and so forth. Each training session started with a joke of the day and the reading of funny stories. Participants were shown how to give priority to humour in their everyday lives and were taught laughing exercises and games as well as being encouraged to share their own funny stories. At the end of the last session, participants shared their portfolios with one another. Researchers found that participants reported a decrease in pain and perception of loneliness as well as an increase in life satisfaction and happiness. Similarly, Kugler and colleagues (2021) designed one-hour training sessions (once a week for four weeks) that aimed to encourage people who lived with persistent pain to express joy and cheerfulness, to allow themselves to laugh and to give humour more space in their everyday lives. They were also taught about what humour could do and were encouraged to take part in creative, practical exercises to help them look at situations from a more humorous point of view. The participants said they mostly enjoyed the sessions. In terms of the measures taken before and after, although their depression and cheerfulness levels stayed the same, there was a trend for better quality of life and reduced pain intensity.

I am really interested to learn more about which elements made the most difference in the humour training. In both the studies not only were the participants being taught to actively look for the positive each day, but they were also meeting once a week with other people and so were socialising. I wonder whether attending training with others in a similar situation was actually more important than the training itself in terms of the improvements that were reported? In completing training that was designed to be fun, creative, and funny, participants were given the opportunity to laugh with others and increase their social circle. Was it learning to reframe their perspective that made the difference, and/or was it meeting with others who were also actively looking for the positive? After all, if we focus on the negative, that is what we see; similarly, looking for funny things will help us see the funny side. This sounds like an interesting area to keep an eye on.

Clown doctors

In reading the literature for this chapter, I learned that there are such things as medical clowns. Their role is to turn a patient's experience into something more tolerable. Karnieli-Miller and colleagues (2023) explain that clown doctors say the things that they imagine a patient might want to say, but not feel able to. For example, when a patient has just finished a physiotherapy exercise, the clown asks 'That's it. Is he done? Only one more exercise left?' and the therapist confirms there is indeed one more exercise. The clown then replies with disappointment and surprise that there is indeed 'another exercise'. In doing this, the clown is voicing what the patient finds hard to say. The clowning is described as an art form that invites play, interaction and laughter (Tan et al., 2014). Clown doctors or hospital clowns are professional artists who complete a rigorous training programme before they are allowed to work in a hospital setting (Dionigi et al., 2025). Their task is to bring play, humour, and laughter to the patient and their family members, as well as to the hospital staff. They focus on 'transforming the care setting into a more uplifting environment' (Dionigi et al., 2025, p. 2).

Clown care has been shown to help reduce anxiety and fear in hospitalised children, lessen their post-operative pain, and have a positive impact on the children's health outcomes as they recover from their disease (Ding et al., 2022; Xin et al., 2024). Clown care can also bring lightness to serious situations: for example, a parent in Tan and colleagues' study of clown care in a Finnish children's hospital (2014, p. 5) said that clown care 'helped relax the atmosphere when something frightening comes or is happening to the child'. However, clowns are not liked by everyone, and some people (children and adults) are afraid of them. (In case you are interested, the name for having a phobia of clowns is 'coulrophobia'.) For this reason, Tan and colleagues (2014) concluded that, although clown care can bring benefits, better understanding is needed of when it is and, more importantly, when it is not appropriate to introduce clown care. Drawing similar conclusions, a more recent review by Xin et al (2024) showed that although clown care had a number of benefits (including alleviating children's worries and distracting them from their illness), not all hospitalised children benefitted from clown care.

What about adults and clown care?

Given most of the studies exploring clown care have focused on children, Dionigi and Canestrari (2016) pose the question 'How do clown interventions affect adults within the hospital setting?'. They highlighted a study by Brutsche and colleagues (2008) that evaluated the effect of laughter induced by a clown in a group of patients with chronic obstructive pulmonary disease (COPD). Pello the clown had been asked to make the group laugh as much as possible in the half hour he was interacting with them. Although this was a small sample, the findings showed an improvement in the lung function of the experimental group.

But what about persistent pain: Can clown care help with that?

In terms of clown care and pain, there are two recent reviews of the published literature. Lopes-Júnior and colleagues (2020) reviewed studies evaluating the effect of hospital clowns during the use of invasive, painful, anxiety-inducing medical procedures and concluded that hospital clown interventions helped to relieve the pain and emotional distress in children undergoing these painful and stressful procedures. Ding and colleagues (2022) also reviewed the research and concluded that clown interventions could be a promising way to relieve acute pain in children.

Clown care is not, as yet, something that has been widely explored with adult populations, nor with people who are living with persistent pain. So, for the purposes of this book, clown doctors are an interesting thing to know about, but not (yet) relevant to helping us live well with chronic pain. This might make you feel a little annoyed. Conveniently, we are about to turn our attention to swearing.

SWEARING

I first came across the idea that swearing might be useful for pain when I was working in a pain management clinic and was reading as much of the research literature as I could to make sure I was up to date with current thinking. I remember reading a paper entitled; 'Swearing as a response to pain'. The authors (Stephens, Atkins, and Kingston, 2009) had noticed that swearing was a common response to pain, and they were interested in exploring whether swearing made any difference to the experience of pain. They did not set out to explore persistent pain, but instead wondered whether swearing might impact our tolerance for pain.

What is swearing?

Swearing is what we do when we use specific, negative, and often emotional words, which are taboo and so are very likely to cause offence (Beers Fägersten, 2012). In 1901 Professor G. Patrick from the University of Iowa wrote a paper called 'The Psychology of Profanity' (1901). He was exploring the questions: 'Why do men swear?' and 'When they swear, why do they use the words which they do?'. He concluded that swearing was a primitive and instinctive reaction to a situation that a person felt threatened their wellbeing. Vingerhoets and colleagues (2013, p. 288) suggest that humans have been 'using curse and swear words since the emergence of language'. For example, they referred to the punishments for swearing in the fifteenth century, which included being imprisoned, having one's tongue cut out, and even the death penalty. Patrick (1901, p. 117) stated that swearing 'still widely prevails throughout the world, especially among soldiers and sailors, in the laboring classes, among the uneducated and among criminals'. This view of who swears has changed a lot. Indeed, Washmuth and Stephens (2022) note that the assumption that swearing is a masculine activity is no longer correct. (As an aside, I know this is very juvenile of me and I am sure I am not the first to say something about this, but I love that a person called 'Washmuth' is a swearing researcher. Their name is not so far away from what people who swore at school were told to do: to go and wash their mouth (Washmuth) out with soap.) Vingerhoets and colleagues (2013) suggest that, nowadays, women tend to swear as much or even more often than men (see, for example, the work of Johnson and Lewis, 2010; Stone and Hazelton, 2008).

Swear words have the 'potential to be offensive, inappropriate, objectionable or unacceptable in any given context' (Beers Fägersten, 2012, p. 3). However, Stapleton and colleagues (2022) note that it can be hard to pin down exact definitions and criteria for swearing. The list of what counts as a swear word is also likely to vary culturally and at different points in time. For example, Eileen Finn (2017) was considering how or, indeed, whether to include swearing when she was teaching English as a second language. She writes: 'understanding that swear words have different levels of offensiveness is pertinent in being able to identify verbal aggression. Moreover, students are disconnected from swear words because they do not have the same impact as they would on a native speaker' (Finn, 2017, p. 21). A great example of just such a scenario is reported by Stapleton and colleagues (2022) who share the example of a British tennis player who had been playing in an Italian competition. When interviewed, she was asked whether she had learned any Italian. She shared a phrase her friend had taught her, and could tell by the shocked faces of the interviewing team that the phrase was unlikely to be a polite one.

Context is important. For example, Lev-Ari and McKay (2022, p. 1103) share what to me is a light-hearted example, though to science fiction enthusiasts it is likely a very serious example. The authors note: 'Aficionados of Star Wars, Star Trek and Battlestar Galactica know that the words "fierfek", "grozit" and "frak" are not to be used in polite company.' I am not familiar with these films, but I can understand from that contextual sentence that, were I to utter any of these phrases, I would likely cause offence if I was in the presence of other speakers of these different languages. So we need to be able to understand swear words and the context for their use, not just if we want to use them ourselves, but also to ensure that we are correctly interpreting what it is another person is trying to tell us.

An interesting question is why, when we have such an amazing array of words to choose from, do we resort to swearing. In answer to this, Stapleton and colleagues (2022, p. 2) note that 'swearing is powerful'. Some studies have shown that when we swear we feel that we can release or express negative emotions more clearly (see, for example, Baruch et al., 2017, who explored swearing at work). Interestingly, for people who speak more than one language, swearing in their first language is felt to have a greater emotional intensity than swearing in languages learned later in life (see, for example, Shakiba and Stapleton (2022) who studied Persian immigrants' language choice for swearing).

What are the impacts of swearing?

Hay and colleagues (2024) mentioned the positive physiological, psychological, and social effects of swearing. They reported that swearing can improve physical performance, increase self-confidence, increase humour, improve credibility, and strengthen social connections. Swearing can be an expression of joy or excitement. There is, of course, a caveat that this is very much context dependent. Think here about the formality of the situation, the swearing tolerance of those nearby, social and cultural expectations, and so forth. However, we often think of swearing as being associated with the release of negative emotions (e.g., anger and frustration), or perhaps as a way of insulting other people or as a way of making an insult even stronger. In other words, it can be used with the intent to cause offence, as an 'impoliteness strategy' (Stapleton et al., 2022, p. 7). In short there is a whole world of research exploring the positive and negative effects of swearing. Researchers have explored what makes some words taboo, why some words feel more satisfying to say than others, what the function is of swearing, whether it helps us to bond with others, and what might be the cultural, biological, social, and psychological influences on swearing. However, we will be looking at one small (but extremely important for us), aspect of the swearing evidence. Can swearing have a positive impact on pain?

So what is it about swearing and pain? Some researchers have suggested that part of the power of swearing comes from the way the words sound when you say them. Indeed, Patrick (1901, pp. 117–118) suggested that even people who do not usually swear can find some words very satisfying to say when they are feeling annoyed or frustrated. He gives the example of struggling to do up a collar button, and how the frustration experienced can be released by saying the word 'Damn' emphatically. He suggests: 'the word seems to have been made for the occasion.' Continuing with this theme, Lev-Ari and McKay (2022) were interested in learning whether the sound of swear words was important. They noted that, in common with animals, we humans make harsh, spiky sounds when we are distressed and smooth sounds when we feel calm. Given this tendency, they wondered whether there are some sounds that are perfect for swear words. They asked native Hebrew, Hindi, Hungarian, Korean, and Russian speakers to provide a list of five to ten of the most vulgar words in their language that were used when someone got hurt or was frustrated, as well as the most offensive words that were used to insult someone. They then did some complicated linguistic things that enabled them to work out the most common sounds in these swear words. From this, they developed false words that they could use in their study. Participants who took part were told they would hear pairs of words in different languages and that their job was to identify the swear word in each pair. What they did not know was that all the words in the pairs were made up words. I am oversimplifying what was a complex study here, but the authors concluded that some sounds were indeed more likely to be considered appropriate for swearing.

So can swearing help us tolerate pain?

Obviously, the decision to deliberately cause someone pain just to see whether swearing makes the pain more or less bearable needs careful consideration. We have ethical guidelines as researchers and practitioners to ensure we do no harm. However, there is an experiment called the cold pressor test (CPT) that causes pain in a safe manner. Kiviniemi and colleagues (2011) report that CPTs are generally safe and well tolerated. A person doing the cold pressor test is asked to plunge their hand (though it can be other parts of the body) into cold water. Stephens and colleagues (2009) invited their participants to try swearing to see if this would increase the length of time that they could leave their limb in the cold water.

By way of a bit of extra information, in case you are interested, the cold pressor test was developed by a doctor called Edgar A. Hines so that he could study blood pressure variability (you can read more about the history of this test in the paper by Lamotte et al., 2021). When you put a part of your body in something so cold that it is experienced as painful, there will be an effect on your body. For example, your arteries tighten up, your heart rate increases, and, as a consequence, your blood pressure will rise. This rise in blood pressure is known as the pressor response. So, when Edgar A. Hines induced the pressor response using cold as a trigger, he named his new test the 'cold pressor test'.

I'm guessing you might have a few questions about the cold pressor test. Fanninger and colleagues were interested in how cold the water was in cold pressor tests. They published a paper in 2023 that explored this and other questions. Among 331 trials that they reviewed, they found that the most commonly reported water temperature was 1 degree centigrade. They also reported that, in most of the studies, researchers had pre-set a maximum time that they would let their participants keep their limb(s) in the water. There were two common maximum times: 180 seconds or 300 seconds. Though Fanninger and colleagues (2023) also note that researchers did not always explain whether they told their participants that there was a pre-set maximum time they would be allowed to keep their limb in the water. This is important. I imagine if I was about to do the cold pressor test and I knew that there was a maximum time I would be allowed to keep my limb in the water, I would be tempted to see if I could last the full allotted time. If, on the other hand, the researchers did not mention there was a maximum time that I would be allowed to keep my hand in the water, I might not be so stubborn about trying to beat the clock.

We can focus back now to Richard Stephens and colleagues (2009). Although swearing is a very common response to pain, they wondered whether swearing might alter a person's experience of pain. And so their cold pressor swearing experiment was born. I am oversimplifying what was done but, in essence, people who took part were asked to repeat a swear word or a neutral word while their hand was in the cold water. The researchers timed how long the participants could keep their hand in the cold water. They found that swearing increased pain tolerance.

Incidentally, in 2014 I changed jobs and moved from Bath to Stoke-on-Trent. As a way of getting to know people locally (I knew no one when I made the move), I set up 'Psychology in the Pub'. Once a month, I would invite a psychologist to come to a friendly local pub and share something interesting about their research with whoever happened to be in the pub that evening. I was based at the University of Staffordshire and just up the road was Keele University, which also had a thriving psychology department, and it was where Richard Stephens was based. Of course I invited Richard, and later his excellent PhD student (at that time), Olivia Robertson, to come and give talks on their swearing research. Richard included a quiz in his talk to try to establish who in the pub that evening was the most prone to swearing. It is one of my claims to fame that, thanks to votes from my colleagues, I was identified as being the second most sweary in the pub that night! This aside, there is a downside to being someone who swears often in daily life. Looking over their findings from their first cold pressor swearing study, Stephens and colleagues noticed that there was a small group who were not helped by swearing. So Stephens and Umland (2011) repeated the original experiment, but this time they included the question 'How many times a day do you swear?'. This study showed that those who swore frequently in daily life benefitted less from swearing during the task. In other words, Stephens and Umland (2011, p. 1274) concluded that 'overuse of swearing in everyday settings lessens its effectiveness as a short-term intervention to reduce pain'.

In another study. Stephens and Robertson (2020) explored whether the sound of swear words was important. They created two new swear words to see if they had a similar effect on pain tolerance as real swear words. One of the newly invented swear words was designed to be satisfying to say ('fouch') and the other ('twizpipe') to offer distraction through humour. (As a brief aside, I emailed Richard to ask how to pronounce 'fouch'. I wondered if it rhymed with touch or ouch. He let me know that to pronounce it correctly it should rhyme with 'ouch'.) Stephens and Robertson (2020) used the cold pressor test to trial these new swear words. People taking part had to say the word they were given at a normal speech volume, once every three seconds. The researchers found that although the invented swear words were similar to real swear words in terms of raised emotion and humour ratings, they were not effective at improving pain tolerance. In other words, it seems we need to use real swear words to experience the benefit, and the swear words we use are better if they are words of our own choosing (Stephens et al., 2018).

Is there a place for swearing in clinic?

We already know from Richard Stephens' work that swearing (as long as you do not swear too much in your day-to-day life) can increase your pain tolerance. Washmuth and Stephens (2022, p. 2) suggest that 'swearing can lead to tighter human bonds and create informal environments where people are more likely to be themselves'. They also note that in a physical therapy setting, a positive therapeutic alliance has been linked to improvements in musculoskeletal pain (see, for example, Fuentes et al., 2014; Kinney et al., 2020; Zimney et al., 2025). So, they wondered, could swearing in clinic be useful? Might it strengthen the bond between patient and clinician? Might it help the patient complete the physical therapy exercises? However, swearing is generally viewed as unprofessional (Washmuth et al., 2024). Indeed, most codes of professional conduct will refer to the importance of the careful choice of language to avoid causing offence. Words have the potential to strengthen or weaken the therapeutic alliance and cause either healing or harm. With this in mind, Giffin (2016) surveyed 50 patients who had experienced swearing from their health professional. Eighty per cent of them said this had had a positive impact on their therapeutic relationship. None felt it had

had a negative impact. In contrast, Trummer and colleagues (2023) reported two cases where a physical therapist had used swearing in the clinical setting. One patient felt their social connection with their therapist had improved as a consequence. The other thought it decreased their connection. Neither thought that the swearing was unprofessional. In another study, Washmuth and colleagues (2023) reported a case where a proposal to include swearing had been made in a patient's fourth session with a physiotherapist. The patient was told about the literature showing that swearing might help with pain and she agreed to include it in her session. She chose her swear word and used it during the most painful and challenging physiotherapy exercises in her remaining sessions. She reported finding it funny. She said it provided a distraction from the pain and helped her to feel more confident. While acknowledging that this was just one patient, Washmuth and Stephens (2022) recognise the need to proceed with care to avoid offending patients, whereas Washmuth and colleagues (2023) highlight the potential positive impact that swearing could have in this kind of clinical setting.

SO, IS IT TRUE THAT LAUGHTER AND SWEARING CAN HELP WITH PERSISTENT PAIN?

Most of the research that has been conducted in the humour and swearing fields has focused on acute pain. However, it is clear that laughter and humour have the potential to make us all feel more positive. Being prompted to look actively for the positive can increase our wellbeing. However, whether humour and laughter can impact on the persistent pain experience is not yet clear. With respect to swearing, it seems that it has an effect on our ability to tolerate acute pain (the cold pressor test, which is used to measure pain tolerance, is a test that the participant knows will end – it is a short-term pain, rather than a chronic pain). The swearing improves tolerance for short-term pain but how this works is not yet known. We also know that most people who have completed the cold pressor test have been college age students who were fit and well. So the work on swearing and pain has focused on acute (short-term) pain in controlled laboratory settings. Indeed, Hay and colleagues (2024) are clear that we know much less about the impact of swearing on persistent pain; and Robertson, Robinson, and Stephens (2017, p. 271) recognise that whilst 'transient experimental pain does not replicate the complex and nuanced sensory and affective facets of clinical pain', they hope that this body of work will contribute to better understanding of the pain experience. So, at the moment, we know that humour and laughter improve quality of life, and swearing definitely helps with acute pain – but as for the extent to which these things work for people who live with persistent pain? We do not yet know.

FURTHER RESOURCES

For an exploration of the history of swearing, this is an accessible (and very sweary) book: M. Mohr (2013). *Holy sh*t: A brief history of swearing*. Oxford University Press.

For a very interesting article about swearing, see K. Beers Fägersten (2012). English language swearing as humor in Swedish comic strips. *Journal of Pragmatics*, 121, 175–187.

The Brickworks Museum: https://thebrickworksmuseum.org/ [accessed 7 February 2026].

Dr Kataria's laughter yoga: https://laughteryoga.org/ [accessed 10 January 2026].

REFERENCES

Baruch, Y., Prouska, R., Ollier-Malaterre, A., and Bunk, J. (2017). Swearing at work: The mixed outcomes of profanity. *Journal of Managerial Psychology*, 32(2), 149–162.

Basler, J., Potó, D., Kumli, K., et al. (2025). Why aren't you laughing? The effect of dark and light humour on anxiety and affective state. *Personality and Individual Differences*, 240, 113133. https://www.sciencedirect.com/science/article/pii/S0191886925000959.

Beers Fägersten, K. (2012). *Who's swearing now? The social aspects of conversational swearing*. Cambridge Scholars Publishing.

Bennett, M.P. and Lengacher, C.A. (2006). Humor and laughter may influence health. I. History and background. *Evidence-Based Complementary and Alternative Medicine*, 3(1), 61–63.

Brutsche, M.H., Grossman, P., Müller, R.A., et al. (2008). Impact of laughter on air trapping in severe obstructive lung disease. *International Journal of COPD*, 3(1), 185–192.

Ding, Y., Yin, H., Wang, S., et al. (2022). Effectiveness of clown intervention for pain relief in children: A systematic review and meta-analysis. *Journal of Clinical Nursing*, 31 (21022), 3000–3010.

Dionigi, A. and Canestrari, C. (2016). Clowning in health care settings: The point of view of adults. *Europe's Journal of Psychology*, 12(3), 473–488.

Dionigi, A., Canestrari, C., and Fermani, A. (2025). Caring with humor: How cognitive flexibility enhances humor and playfulness in clown doctors. *Journal of Humanistic Psychology*. https://doi.org/10.1177/00221678251336487.

Fanninger, S., Plener, P., Fischer, M.J.M., and Kothgassner, O.D. (2023). Water temperature during the cold pressor test: A scoping review. *Physiology & Behavior*, 271, 114354. https://doi.org/10.1016/j.physbeh.2023.114354.

Finn, E. (2017). Swearing: The good, the bad & the ugly. *ORTESOL Journal*, 34, 17–26.

Fuentes, J., Armijo-Olivo, S., Funabashi, M., et al. (2014). Enhanced therapeutic alliance modulates pain intensity and muscle pain sensitivity in patients with chronic low back pain: An experimental controlled study. *Physical Therapy*, 94: 477–489.

Giffin, H.J. (2016). *Clients' experiences and perceptions of the therapist's use of swear words and the resulting impact on the therapeutic alliance in the context of the therapeutic relationship*. Master's thesis, Smiths College. Published online 2016. Available at https://scholarworks.smith.edu/cgi/viewcontent.cgi?article=2787&context=theses [accessed 30 January 2026].

Gonot-Schoupinsky, F.N. and Garip, G. (2019). Prescribing laughter to increase well-being in healthy adults: An exploratory mixed method feasibility study of the Laughie. *European Journal of Integrative Medicine*, 26, 56–64. https://www.sciencedirect.com/science/article/pii/S1876382018308977.

Hay, C.M., Sills, J.L., Shoemake, J.M., et al. (2024). F@#$pain! A mini-review of the hypoalgesic effects of swearing. *Frontiers in Psychology*, 15, 1416041.

Johnson, D.I. and Lewis, N. (2010). Perceptions of swearing in the work setting: An expectancy violations theory perspective. *Communication Reports*, 23, 106–118.

Karnielei-Miller, O., Divon-Ophir, O., Sagi, D., et al. (2023). More than just an entertainment show: Identification of medical clowns' communication skills and therapeutic goals. *Qualitative Health Research*, 33(1–2), 25–38.

Kim, B. and Choi, S. (2025). The efficacy of laughter-based interventions in children: A systematic review and meta-analysis. *Journal of Child Health Care*. doi: 10.1177/13674935251346886.

Kinney, M., Seider, J., Beaty, A.F., et al. (2020). The impact of therapeutic alliance in physical therapy for chronic musculoskeletal pain: A systematic review of the literature. *Physiotherapy Theory and Practice*, 36(8), 886–898.

Kiviniemi, T.O., Schindler, T., Tulppo, M., et al. (2011). Cold pressor test safety: The incidence of vasovagal reactions. *American Journal of Cardiology*, 107, 492–493. https://www.sciencedirect.com/science/article/pii/S0002914910021193?via%3Dihub.

Kugler, L., Kuhbandner, C., Gerum, S., et al. (2021). Evaluation of a humor training for patients with chronic pain: A randomized clinical trial. *Journal of Pain Research*, 14, 3121–3133.

Lamotte, G., Boes, C.J., Low, P.A., and Coon, E.A. (2021). The expanding role of the cold pressor test: A brief history. *Clinical Autonomic Research*, 31, 153–155. https://link.springer.com/article/10.1007/s10286-021-00796-4.

Lapierre, S.S., Baker, B.D., and Tanaka, H. (2019). Effects of mirthful laughter on pain tolerance: A randomized controlled investigation. *Journal of Bodywork and Movement Therapies*, 23, 733–738.

Lev-Ari, S. and McKay, R. (2022). The sound of swearing: Are there universal patterns in profanity? *Psychonomic Bulletin & Review*, 30, 1103–1114.

Lopes-Júnior, L., Bomfim, E., Olson, K., et al. (2020). Effectiveness of hospital clowns for symptom management in paediatrics: Systematic review of randomised and non-randomised controlled trials. *BMJ*, 371, m4290.

Patrick, G.T.W. (1901). The psychology of profanity. *The Psychological Review*, 3(2), 113–127.

Robertson, O., Robinson, S.J., and Stephens, R. (2017). Swearing as a response to pain: A cross-cultural comparison on British and Japanese participants. *Scandinavian Journal of Pain*, 17, 267–272.

Shakiba, N. and Stapleton, K. (2022). Persian immigrants' language choice for swearing: The effects of socio-biographical variables and personality traits. *Journal of Multilingual and Multicultural Development*, 1–18. https://www.tandfonline.com/doi/full/10.1080/01434632.2022.2068559.

Sharma, A., Singh, M., and Gusain, V.J. (2024). The philosophical basis and significance of laughter yoga: Examining its association to mindfulness, positive psychology and overall well-being. *International Journal of Applied Research*. https://doi.org/10.22271/allresearch.2024.v10.i3a.11572.

Spytska, L. (2024). Effect of laughter therapy on the psychological and physiological state of a person. *Psichologija*, 71, 118–132.

Stapleton, K., Fägersten, K.B., Stephens, R., and Loveday, C. (2022). The power of swearing: What we know and what we don't. *Lingua*. https://doi.org/10.1016/j.lingua.2022.103406.

Stephens, R. and Robertson, O. (2020). Swearing as a response to pain: Assessing hypoalgesic effects of novel 'swear' words. *Frontiers in Psychology*, 11, 723. doi: 10.3389/fpsyg.2020.00723.

Stephens, R., Atkins, J., and Kingston, A. (2009). Swearing as a response to pain. *NeuroReport*, 20(12), 1056–1060.

Stephens, R., Spierer, D.K., and Katehis, E. (2018). Effect of swearing on strength and power performance. *Psychology of Sport and Exercise*, 35, 111–117.

Stephens, R. and Umland, C. (2011). Swearing as a response to pain: Effect of daily swearing frequency. *The Journal of Pain*, 12(12), 1274–1281.

Stone, T.E. and Hazelton, M. (2008). An overview of swearing and its impact on mental health nursing practice. *International Journal of Mental Health Nursing*, 17, 208–214.

Tan, A.K., Eija, M., and Hannula, L. (2014). Benefits and barriers of clown care: A qualitative phenomenological study of parents with children in clown care services. *European Journal of Humour research*, 2(2) 1–10.

Trummer, G., Stephens, R., and Washmuth, N.B. (2023). A physical therapist who swears: A case series. *Journal of Clinical Rehabilitation Medicine*, 6, jmcc 010277.

Tse, M.M.Y., Lo, A.P.K., Cheng, T.L.Y., et al. (2010). Humor therapy: Relieving chronic pain and enhancing happiness for older adults. *Journal of Aging Research*. https://doi.org/10.4061/2010/343574.

Vingerhoets, A.J.J.M., Bylsma, L.M., and de Vlam, C. (2013). Swearing: A biopsychosocial perspective. *Psychological Topics*, 22 (2), 287–304.

Warren, C., Barksy, A., and McGraw, A.P. (2021). What makes things funny? An integrative review of the antecedents of laughter and amusement. *Personality and Social Psychology Review*, 25(1), 41–65.

Washmuth, N.B., Meakins, A., Trummer, G., and Stephens, R. (2024). Can swearing be professional and patient-centred? *Journal of Humanities in Rehabilitation*. https://www.jhrehab.org/2024/04/12/can-swearing-be-professional-and-patient-centered/.

Washmuth, N.B. and Stephens, R. (2022). Frankly, we do give a damn: Improving patient outcomes with swearing. *Archives of Physiotherapy*, 12, 6. https://doi.org/10.1186/s40945-022-00131-8.

Washmuth, N.B., Stephens, R., McAfee, B., et al. (2023). Using expletives to enhance therapeutic outcomes: A case report. *Health Psychology Research*, 11 (1). https://doi.org/10.52965/001c.89726.

Xin, G., Yingping, F., Yue, C., et al. (2024). Application of clown care in hospitalised children: A scoping review. *PloS One*, 19(12), e0313841.

Zimney, K.J., Puentedura, E., Kolber, M.J., and Louw, A. (2025). The correlation of trust as part of the therapeutic alliance in physical therapy and their relation to outcomes for patients with chronic low back pain. *Physiotherapy Theory and Practice*, 41(3), 471–480.

6

WHAT HAS PSYCHOLOGY GOT TO DO WITH PERSISTENT PAIN?

INTRODUCTION

People who live with persistent pain are faced with many challenges. They often have a long journey to diagnosis and, along the way, have to navigate a complex health system that is not set up for long-term conditions. They will likely face people (health professionals as well as friends, family, and employers) who may not be convinced about the seriousness of their pain. They may have multiple tests to try to identify the cause of their pain. While all this goes on, they may well be prescribed pain medication. However, Wang and colleagues (2025, p. 1) note that many people who are living with persistent pain 'do not achieve clinically significant pain relief through medication alone'. A meta-analysis by Welsch and colleagues (2020) found that people who took opioid pain medication only had marginal improvements to their pain intensity compared to those who were taking a placebo. In other words, although pain medication is often the most common approach for people who live with persistent pain (Wang et al., 2025), medication alone is rarely sufficient. Other approaches (depending on the individual) may also usefully be offered in tandem with, or perhaps instead of, pain medication. Working with a psychologist is one such approach.

DOI: 10.4324/9781003649854-6

Professor Rona Moss-Morris (2013) wrote that coping with a chronic condition was an ongoing process that would never be fully achieved. In saying this, she was acknowledging that, as with everything in life, chronic conditions do not simply arrive, they change with our changing circumstances. This means that coping strategies and health behaviours will also need to change as individuals' lives unfold. In this chapter, I explain how psychology and psychologists can work as part of a multidisciplinary team to help people live well in spite of their pain condition.

WHAT IS PSYCHOLOGY?

Reber (1995, p. 617) wrote: 'Psychology simply cannot be defined; indeed, it cannot even be easily characterized.' However, at its simplest, psychology is the study of the relationship between mind and behaviour. It is about what people think as well as what they do, and how they react to things. And since how we think about things (our beliefs about health and illness), what we do (our health behaviours), and how we react to things (our emotional response) all have a role to play in living well in spite of persistent pain, psychology has a role to play in supporting those who live with persistent pain. This role spans the whole experience of living with persistent pain; from the time that someone begins their journey to diagnosis, and is faced with coping with all the uncertainty, through to accepting the diagnosis and adapting to what this means for them. In addition, people who live with persistent pain often need to change their behaviour if they are to live well in spite of their pain. Psychologists can support behaviour change and can also help increase people's understanding of persistent pain. This increased understanding is really helpful when someone is trying to change a behaviour. Each of these elements are considered in the next section of this chapter.

JOURNEY TO DIAGNOSIS

Health professionals have a key role to play in the patient's journey to diagnosis. In a paper by Dupont and colleagues (2025), both patients and physicians were interviewed. The GPs were concerned about patient expectations and how to manage them. Patients (not surprisingly) wanted to be pain free whereas GPs felt that complete absence of pain was not a realistic goal:

> So I do talk to people about how they unfortunately cannot expect to be completely free of pain, but that the goal is to get them to a level of pain that is as low as possible, but that they can still cope with it in their everyday lives.
>
> (Dupont et al., 2025, p. 9)

In a different study, this time exploring the experiences of trainee doctors who have worked with people living with medically unexplained symptoms, the inability to cure a person was in itself a challenge to the trainees' view of their role: 'In medical school you're taught that patients have things wrong with them and there's always a medical cause for it and you've got to try and find it' (Howman et al., 2016, p. 7). So not only are health professionals faced with working with conditions that they cannot fix, they are also faced with having to explain to patients (who want to be fixed) that there is no cure. This frustration about not being able to help, can result in the health professional becoming short-tempered with the patient. One doctor said: 'I could find myself getting really agitated with him and getting cross as well … I've got lots of other things to do. I don't have time for this' (Howman et al., 2016, p. 9). The experience of the patient is all but forgotten in this quote. The focus is all on the impact on the health professional, with a strong hint of blame about how the patient is somehow wasting the time of the health professional. Their frustration at the situation becomes directed towards the patient, which can in turn lead to labelling of patients. In this example, the health professional was talking about patients living with medically unexplained symptoms (MUS): 'Although we come across them in our training, they are often labelled as heartsink, and no real advice given as to how best help such patients' (Howman et al., 2016, p. 4). This feeling of impotence goes against the training ethos instilled in health professionals: 'There is something quite nice about being able to say, Oh you've got epigastric pain, yes you're

H pylori positive, I can do something about it. You kind of want to fix it don't you' (Howman et al., 2016, p. 5).

The complex technical language used by the interviewee above positions them as expert. This expertise is part of what is 'quite nice', they are the 'all powerful' fixer. Except that with persistent pain it cannot be fixed, just managed. This is difficult to accept:

> The last thing you want to do is leave your patients in pain. It would be lovely if I could get rid of her pain, then all she had to deal with is the rest of her life. Realistically a large proportion of it we can't actually fix.
>
> (Howman et al., 2016, p. 5)

This means that just as health professionals are faced with uncertainty throughout their journey, so too are those who are living every day with the uncertainty of their pain. Gibson and colleagues (2023, p. 2) highlighted that 'long-term conditions often require adjustment and acceptance of ongoing avoidable unknowns'. They go on to make the case that a person's ability to deal with uncertainty is important in the context of living with the long-term conditions. How a person comes to terms with uncertainty impacts on the way they react to their changed reality. This involves how they think (cognitive response), feel (emotional response), and act (behavioural response).

LEARNING

For those who live with persistent pain, it may seem strange to be told that they may benefit from being taught about persistent pain. After all, they live it. They feel it. Every single day. They may well wonder what there is to learn. However, gaining greater insight into and understanding of persistent pain, as well as how experience of and reaction to our pain might be influenced by other things, can be useful. With this extra knowledge, the person with pain may learn new coping strategies that make a positive difference to their experience.

Whilst psychologists are very well placed to provide this teaching, they may face a considerable challenge before they will be listened to. Psychologists can be viewed in a negative way by people who live with pain. The person who is living with pain may be unsure about why they have been referred to psychology. They may be anxious in case the referral is a sign that someone was thinking that their pain was all in their mind. This is not surprising – as has already been mentioned in earlier chapters of this book, too many people who live with persistent pain have been told that the problem is all in their heads. Women in the studies that were reviewed by Biring and colleagues (2025) reported feeling that health professionals had dismissed, rejected, or ignored them when they sought help for their persistent pain. Others felt their pain was trivialised and not taken seriously. By way of example, one participant in a study by Caton and colleagues (2024, p. 1214) said: 'a lot of doctors said that it was in my head'; and another said: 'I was told by doctors, [...] "Oh you're just having bad cramps." It's just like, "No, I know my body, this is not bad cramps".'

Having your own explanation ignored or belittled by the people you turn to for help, and then being told that your symptoms are all in your head, is awful. So it is not surprising that GPs said that they were wary of mentioning psychology to patients living with persistent pain (Dupont et al., 2025). The GPs were afraid that their patients might misinterpret the suggestion of a referral to psychology and assume the GP believed their pain to be psychosomatic. On one hand I can see why a GP might think this. However, a GP has an important role to play in how they share their thinking. Simply suggesting their patient would benefit from seeing a psychologist will quite likely result in the patient assuming the GP thinks their pain is all in the mind. However, the GP could take a little time to explain that how we think and feel can impact on how we behave, and that, in turn, how we behave can be helpful or unhelpful when we are faced with living with persistent pain. If, at that point, the GP then explains that psychologists are trained in understanding the link between thoughts, feelings, and behaviour, and so may be able to help the patient learn new ways to cope with their persistent pain, then perhaps a referral to a psychologist will be seen in a more positive light. We cannot afford for our GPs to be uncomfortable about referring patients to psychologists.

A psychologist who is trained in pain management will be able to explain why therapies that are not directly focused on the body itself can make a positive difference, not least because it reassures the patient that they are not, as they once feared, going 'barmy':

> It [education programme] also reassured me that I wasn't going barmy [...] it explained that I'm not. What I am experiencing is real and it explained why, without something necessarily being wrong [...] things like the sensitivity is a kind of new thing that no one had offered before [Participant B, after completing education programme].
>
> (Moseley et al., 2025, p. 4)

As you learn more about your persistent pain, you also understand more about the ways in which different things might impact on your pain experience. This means that when a psychologist works with you to plan how you can change a behaviour, it makes more sense to you. You begin to see how things are linked together and that changing one can have a positive impact on another. Butler and Moseley (2018, p. 11) summarised this process when they said:

> Even when pain is chronic and nasty, it hurts because the brain has concluded for some reason or another, that you are threatened and in danger and need protecting. The trick is finding out why the brain has come to this conclusion.

ACCEPTANCE

Accepting the life-changing nature of living with persistent pain is not straightforward. After all, pain impacts on all aspects of a person's life. Some of the things that they used to be able to do without thinking are now very difficult or perhaps impossible. In their review of the literature focusing on women's experiences of living with persistent pain, Biring and colleagues (2025, p. 38) quoted participants from different studies who said: 'The pain takes over, there is nothing except pain and work' (Hallberg & Carlsson, 1998). Another said it impacted 'everything in everyday life. It limits me in my roles as a mother, wife, cook, friend ... put a stop to ambitions and goals' (Hervik et al., 2023). Indeed, as the pain takes up more space, the person living with pain experiences a series of losses. Charmaz (1983, p. 168), in her paper entitled 'Loss of Self: A Fundamental Form of Suffering in the Chronically Ill', wrote about how people living with long-term conditions often: 'experience a crumbling away of their former self-images without simultaneous development of equally valued new ones. The experiences and meanings upon which these ill persons had built former positive self-images are no longer available to them.' This is, in effect, the start of the process of saying goodbye to your imagined future. After all, we all make assumptions about what our future might look like and so, when we develop something that not only gets in the way of our plans but completely derails them, it is a big shock. In the review by Biring and colleagues (2025), the loss of the life that people had hoped for was spoken of. In a study by Osborn and Smith (1998, p. 70), a participant captured this feeling when they said:

> I'm only 50 and I should be doing this, that and the other cos they say life begins at 40 but I can't. And I s'pose it does bother me. It's frustrating that people of my own age are ... and you feel as though you can't.

It takes time to be able to face up to this new reality. It is not surprising that people need to be able to express their dismay at what has happened. As they learn more about persistent pain (and just how many people are living with it), they move from 'Why me?' towards a more accepting 'Why not me?'. The ultimate goal being to come to terms with the understanding that this is a long-term condition. This is summed up by a participant who took part in a study by Herbert and colleagues (2025, p. 3) who said:

> Pain is there but I don't count it as my enemy; more my friend. I just count it as something to just be dealt with; to be managed without it taking over my life. My life still needs to go on even through the pain. I don't stop enjoying life because of it.

The person in the quote above is able to explore who they are now, and who they can be now that they recognise themselves as a person who lives with persistent pain. In a study exploring women's experiences of living with chronic headaches, Hervik and colleagues (2023, p. 706) report that loss of identity and grief for their former selves were themes mentioned by many of their participants. For example, Mona felt she was a duller version of her previous self. She said she had 'lost myself, somewhere. My identity – gone, washed away by pain and illness. I don't know how to find myself again'. The pain was seen as changing who they were, and this change was not for the better. Katrine said she had: 'become another version of myself. I have become somewhat egocentric; I don't want to be like that. I feel like I have become distant, like I am looking at myself from afar.' Others spoke of hiding the depths of their pain for fear of worrying their loved ones. This is clear in the quote from Rose: 'I am ashamed of being useless, so I pretend, to protect them, and retain some degree of dignity, even though it is false.' These quotes are really quite difficult to read; the harshness with which they judge themselves and the resultant shame is palpable. There is a clear role for psychology here, to help people with persistent pain navigate this life-changing diagnosis. For example, acceptance and commitment therapy (often shortened to ACT) is increasingly offered through pain management programmes. ACT is a therapeutic approach that focuses on developing what is called 'psychological flexibility' (see McCracken, 2023). Psychological flexibility allows us to 'engage in valued activities while being mindfully aware and accepting of whatever internal experiences are present' (Klimczak et al., 2023, p. 271).

One way of achieving this is to acknowledge the pain but focus on living life to the full. For example, a participant in a study by Herbert and colleagues (2025, p. 3) said he can:

> acknowledge that it's there, you know, 'I see you, you're there, and I validate you', and just let go. And, try to stay in the present moment and just recognize that I'm not going to allow it to take over.

Others in the same study spoke of how they focused on reducing the power of their pain. Participant 18 said: 'It's just going to be part of my life, but it's not going to rule my life.' There was an awareness that pain would take as much space as it could, and that part of acceptance was recognising the existence of pain, and then focusing on your own life. Participant 29 said: 'My pain is still there. I don't think it's honestly ever going to go away. So [I am] just accepting it for what it is, and not allowing it to determine my life.' Similar experiences were reported by people who had been given 12 months access to a digital pain self-management programme (see Strand et al., 2025). Participants in this study said that the programme had helped them revise their view of their pain in such a way that they were able to take a more relaxed and optimistic attitude towards their future. For example, one participant said:

> You shouldn't get stuck if you're troubled with some chronic pain, it's actually possible to learn to live with it. Yes. That you can make everyday life better. Yeah. I have accepted it a bit more (...). Then I do not feel down as much, if you know what I mean. I adapt my everyday life more now, based on how the day is going (ID 53).
>
> (Strand et al., 2025, p. 6)

Helping people who live with persistent pain work towards acceptance of this life-changing diagnosis is therefore something psychologists can offer. In this section I have focused on two studies both of whom have implemented ACT as a therapeutic approach. There is a growing body of evidence highlighting the success of this approach for people living with persistent pain (see McCracken et al., 2022; NICE, 2021; Scott & McCracken, 2015).

BEHAVIOUR CHANGE

When you live with persistent pain, your behaviour might change gradually over time. For example, Cheung and colleagues (2025, p. 10) looked at lots of papers reporting the experiences of older adults who were living with persistent pain. They noticed that participants found it challenging to interact with people who did not understand persistent pain. To cope with this, they would shut down conversations. For example, one person said: 'When people ask me how I was doing, I always say I am fine.' Alternatively, they removed themselves from social situations, preferring instead, to be alone: 'I already had my fun, and now I'd rather stay home and not bother anyone. I try to avoid it [socialising] at all costs.' Although this seems like a protective coping strategy, the trouble with avoiding people and invitations is that your life begins to shrink.

Maybe pain-related behaviour change happens as a direct result of the impact of pain on your mobility. Perhaps this means that you are no longer able to take part in your favourite sport. Maybe you cannot drive your car any more. Maybe you cannot play 'rough and tumble' with your children. Maybe behaviour change involves bringing in new things. Perhaps your physiotherapist recommends you exercise daily. Maybe you will be prescribed medication that needs to be taken at specific times in the day. Adding new things into our routine can be difficult. We all have regular habits. A common part of your morning routine is very likely to be toothbrushing (why is it called 'toothbrushing' and not 'teethbrushing'?). Perhaps you clean your teeth morning and evening and you do this because it is just what you do. It has become an automatic habit – something you have done every day for years. You do not even need to think about it anymore. In contrast, adding in new things to our routines sounds easy (after all the exercises will only take 20 minutes to do), but in reality changing our routines is often difficult to achieve. This difficulty is not always understood by the health professionals who have recommended the behaviour change. For example, Campbell and colleagues (2001) explored why some patients do not do their physiotherapy exercises. They found that although participants in their study understood why they should do their exercises, many only managed to do the exercises that they felt would more easily fit into their everyday life, or were those they felt would bring them the most benefit.

Anyone who has tried to start a new behaviour knows how difficult it is to do, even when you understand the reasons for the need for behaviour change. More recently, Vaikar and Swaminathan (2026) have reviewed the evidence to try to better understand what influences whether people with persistent pain do their home exercises. They concluded that there were lots of things that influenced this particular behaviour. In the short term, whether or not someone would do the exercises was based on how positive a view the patient had of physiotherapy and how much of an obligation they felt towards their therapist. In the longer term, whether or not some carried on doing the exercises depended on their symptoms, how easy it was to build the exercises into their lifestyle, their motivation, and whether they felt the exercises were making a difference.

Psychologists are well placed to work with people who need to make changes to their behaviour. We (I am a psychologist, remember!) take into account the person's health beliefs. In other words, we are interested in the story they tell that explains how they have come to live with persistent pain. We want to understand their view of the recommended behaviour change. Do they believe it will help them? And we also want to know whether they think they have the resources (skills, knowledge, ability, time) to put the behaviour change recommendation into practice. Psychologists will also work collaboratively with the person with pain to make sure recommendations fit that person's life context.

HOW MIGHT PSYCHOLOGISTS WORK COLLABORATIVELY WITH SOMEONE WHO HAS PERSISTENT PAIN?

In the health psychology world, colleagues have developed a behaviour change framework that is being successfully used for many different health behaviours. This framework is known as the COM-B model. The letters stand for 'capability', 'opportunity', and 'motivation'. All three of these things are said to be needed if a person is going to be able to successfully change their behaviour ('B'). The model might seem deceptively simple, but it has been built after years of painstaking research by Michie and colleagues (2011). I summarise the different elements of the model below.

- **Capability** is both physical and psychological. In other words, someone who is capable, has the skills and knowledge to make the change in behaviour. Hart and colleagues (2023, p. 8) sum this up as: 'I know it. I know how to do it and I can show how to do it.'
- **Opportunity** is both physical and social. A person who has the opportunity has time, funding, the right equipment, and comes from a culture, or has people round them, who support the proposed behaviour change. Hart and colleagues (2023, p. 8) sum this up as: 'I have everything I need to do it and people whose opinion I care about think I should do it.'
- **Motivation** is described as being both reflective and automatic. Reflective motivation is when you think about the pros and cons of the behaviour. You might be weighing up how difficult the behaviour is going to be, or maybe you will be thinking about whether the effort you will have to make will be worth it in the end. Automatic motivation is more about how you feel emotionally about doing it: your wants and needs. Hart and colleagues (2023, p. 9) sum this up as: 'On balance I think this is a good idea. It is part of my usual practice, it makes me feel good and I just do it without really thinking too much about it.'

This framework is really helpful for giving structure to conversations between a person living with persistent pain and their psychologist. It is important to learn as much as we can about the life context of the person who lives with persistent pain. In a previous book (Rodham, 2020), I used the term 'collaborment'. I define this as a process that brings together collaboration and pain management. When we work in collaborment, we recognise that when you live with persistent pain there are things you can do for yourself, but no one can manage solely by themselves. Collaborment recognises that our life context impacts on our ability to cope. Collaborment recognises that the person with pain brings expertise that complements the expertise held by health professionals. Collaborment also recognises that the person with pain has the right to make informed decisions about how they live their life and how they choose to manage their pain.

So, a psychologist working in collaborment with a person who lives with persistent pain will work to find out as much as they can about that person's 'capability', 'opportunity', and 'motivation'. We could take examples from a paper by Francis and colleagues (2018) that explored the experiences of people who were living with more than one long-term condition. Each person described in the study had been unfairly labelled 'non-compliant' (a horrible term, but one that is commonly used). Diane who lived with arthritis, asthma, and cancer, was unable to manage the exercise machines at a hospital rehabilitation group she had been asked to attend for her asthma. The reason she struggled with the machines was because of her severe arthritis. She simply stopped attending. No one contacted her to find out what had happened. Instead, the rehabilitation group leader wrote to Diane's GP to inform them that Diane was 'non-compliant'. Two other people described in the paper struggled to get to hospital clinics because they could not afford the cost of travel and their responsibilities as carers made it difficult to leave their home for prolonged periods of time. They too were labelled non-compliant. Another example was offered in this paper where a person had explained to a hospital doctor the conflicting priorities that had that impacted on their ability to attend appointments, to which the hospital doctor responded: 'Well, if you don't think your health is important [...].' These scenarios would be potentially avoidable if time was taken with each person to understand their life context. After all, each person in these examples had the motivation to attend rehabilitation or appointments.

Diane had some capability, in that she knew what she needed to do, but she was unable to do it because of her arthritis. In other words, her opportunity was affected. She had motivation, but this was thwarted by the challenges to her opportunity. The exercises she had been prescribed for her asthma were impossible for her to do because of her arthritis. The others had the motivation and capability to get to the appointments (they wanted to attend, they knew how to get there, and they had the skills to do so). What they also lacked was the opportunity. One person did not have sufficient income to be able to afford the cost of travel to the appointments. The other had responsibilities as a carer and so lacked the time to get to the appointment. It is possible that they also lacked support in that they were unable to find someone to step in and take on the caring responsibilities, which would have allowed them to attend their own health appointment. The assumption made by the health professional that people who do not attend appointments are simply not prioritising their health, betrays a gap in empathy and understanding. Being unable to see when someone's life context adds challenges to their situation means that interventions will be unlikely to succeed. Instead of chastising or discharging people from rehabilitation and labelling them as non-compliant, a COM-B conversation may prove enlightening and open up opportunities to find a way together that will help the person concerned help themselves. Someone who is helped to maximise their capability, opportunity, and motivation will develop the competence and confidence to make the changes to their behaviour that in turn could have a positive impact on their ability to live well with their persistent pain.

SO WHAT HAS PSYCHOLOGY GOT TO DO WITH PERSISTENT PAIN?

I hope that this chapter has shown that psychology has a lot to do with persistent pain. And it is not anything to do with someone somewhere thinking that the pain a person is experiencing is imaginary or 'all in their head'. Persistent pain is real and difficult to live with because of the impact it has on all areas of a person's life. For example, stress, anxiety, and worry about our persistent pain and its impact on our life can increase our pain. If we are feeling stressed and anxious, we will likely have trouble thinking straight. Our sleep pattern may be affected (less sleep or too much sleep). Maybe we struggle to do all the things we think we should do, and this feeds into feeling more and more fed up. The things we used to do to cope with our stress have now been taken away from us – maybe we used to run or play sport, but now we cannot. There is much to come to terms with when you live with persistent pain.

Psychologists are able to help the person who lives with persistent pain understand how living with pain impacts on their emotions and mood. Psychologists are also able to explore different skills and behaviours that people with persistent pain can learn that will help them to better cope with the life changes that come when living with persistent pain. Psychologists understand the connection between what we think and feel and how these impact on what we do, and can make use of the COM-B framework as a way of pinpointing areas where the person living with persistent pain might need some extra help. In short, psychologists working with other health professionals in a pain management team can provide an important piece of the puzzle that makes up how a person lives well with persistent pain. In the next chapter, I explore what we can all do to better help those who live with persistent pain to live well, in spite of their persistent pain.

FURTHER RESOURCES

How do I find a psychologist? You could ask your doctor to refer you to a psychologist, or you find your own psychologist. In the United Kingdom, you could use:

Free services

NHS Talking Therapies: You can refer yourself, or ask your GP to refer you. https://www.nhs.uk/nhs-services/mental-health-services/find-nhs-talking-therapies-for-anxiety-and-depression/.

Paid-for services

The British Psychological Society register allows you to find UK psychologists who have chartered status and offer services in your areas. Chartered status is awarded to those psychologists who have reached the highest standard of psychological knowledge and expertise. https://www.bps.org.uk/find-psychologist.

British Association for Counselling and Psychotherapy. https://www.bacp.co.uk/about-therapy/using-our-therapist-directory/

Approved practitioners

When looking for a psychologist, it is important that you check they have the right qualifications and are registered as being able to work as a psychologist. In the United Kingdom, you can check using these websites:

The Health and Care Professions Council (HCPC) register allows you to check that a psychologist is registered as an approved practitioner. https://www.hcpc-uk.org/check-the-register/.

The British Association for Behavioural and Cognitive Psychotherapies (BABCP). If you decide to have cognitive behavioural therapy (CBT) you can check the CBT register. https://portal.babcp.com//therapist/register,

REFERENCES

Biring, S., Burton, A.E., Dunwoody, L., and Kevern, P. (2025). Women's experiences of living with chronic pain: A qualitative meta-synthesis. *British*

Journal of Health Psychology, 30, e70023. https://doi.org/10.1111/bjhp.70023.

Butler, D. and Moseley, L. (2018). *Explain pain*, 2nd edition. Noigroup Publications.

Campbell, R., Evans, M., Tucker, M., et al. (2001). Why don't patients do their exercises? Understanding non-compliance with physiotherapy in patients with osteoarthritis of the knee. *Journal of Epidemiology and Community Health*, 55, 131–138.

Caton, L., Short, N., Goetzinger, A., et al. (2024). 'My goal is ... to get through the day without pain': A qualitative study on chronic pain experiences and treatment needs among child caregiving women. *Maternal and Child Health Journal*, 28, 1210–1218. https://doi.org/10.1007/s10995-024-03915-5.

Charmaz, K. (1983). Loss of self: a fundamental form of suffering in the chronically ill. *Sociology of Health and Illness*, 5(2), 168–195.

Cheung, C.K.C., Cheung, E.T.C., Schoeb, V., et al (2025). Lived experiences of older adults with chronic low back pain and implications on their daily life: A meta-synthesis of qualitative research. *Archives of Rehabilitation Research and Clinical Translation*, 7, 100456. https://doi.org/10.1016/j.arrct.2025.100456.

Dupont, D., Brinkmöller, S., Carter, S., et al. (2025). Exploring physician and patient perspectives on expectations and role models towards chronic pain treatment in general practice: A qualitative cross-sectional study. *Healthcare*, 13, 187. https://doi.org/10.3390/healthcare13020187.

Francis, H., Carryer, J., and Wilkinson, J. (2018). Patient expertise: Contested territory in the realm of long-term condition care. *Chronic Illness*, 15(3), 197–209.

Gibson, B., Rosser, B.A., Schneider, J., and Forshaw, M.J. (2023). The role of uncertainty intolerance in adjusting to long-term physical health conditions: A systematic review. *PLoS ONE*, 18(6), e0286198. https://doi.org/10.1371/journal.pone.0286198.

Hallberg, L.R.-M. and Carlsson, S.G. (1998). Psychosocial vulnerability and maintaining forces related to fibromyalgia: In-depth interviews with twenty-two female patients. *Scandinavian Journal of Caring Sciences*, 12(2), 95–103.

Hart, J., Byrne-Davis, L., Maltinsky, W., and Bull, E. (2023). *Training to change practice: Behavioural science to develop effective health professional education*. Wiley-Blackwell.

Herbert, M.S., Tynan, M., Higdon, A., et al. (2025). Perspectives on an integrated acceptance and commitment therapy and mindfulness meditation program: A qualitative study of veterans with chronic pain. *Journal of Contextual Behavioral Science*, 36, 100885.

Hervik, J.B., Foss, E.B., and Stub, T. (2023). Living with chronic headaches: A qualitative study from an outpatient pain clinic in Norway. *Explore: The Journal of Science and Healing*, 19, 702–709.

Howman, M., Walters, K., Rosenthal, J., et al. (2016). 'You kind of want to fix it don't you?' Exploring general practice trainees' experiences of managing patients with medically unexplained symptoms. *BMC Medical Education*, 16, 27. doi: 10.1186/s12909-015-0523-y.

Klimczak, K.S., San Miguel, G.G., Mukasa, M.N., et al. (2023). A systematic review and meta-analysis of self-guided online acceptance and commitment therapy as a transdiagnostic self-help intervention. *Cognitive Behaviour Therapy*, 52(3), 269–294. https://doi.org/10.1080/16506073.2023.2178498.

McCracken, L.M. (2023). Personalized pain management: Is it time for process-based therapy for particular people with chronic pain? *European Journal of Pain*, 27(9), 1044–1055. https://doi.org/10.1002/ejp.2091.

McCracken, L.M., Yu, L., and Vowles, K. (2022). New generation psychological treatments in chronic pain. *BMJ*, 376, e057212. https //doi.org/10.1136/bmj-2021-057212.

Michie, S., van Stralen, M.M., and West, R. (2011). The behaviour change wheel: A new method for characterising and designing behaviour change interventions. *Implementation Science*, 6, 42.

Moseley, L., Mardon, A., Watson, J., et al. (2025). From didactic explanations to co-design, sequential art and embodied learning: Challenges, criticisms and future directions of patient pain education. *Frontiers in Pain Research*, 6, 1536112. doi: 10.3389/fpain.2025.1536112.

Moss-Morris, R. (2013). Adjusting to chronic illness: Time for a unified theory? *British Journal of Health Psychology*, 18, 681–686.

NICE (2021). Chronic pain (primary and secondary) in over 16s: Assessment of all chronic pain and management of chronic primary pain. *NICE Guideline NG193*. Available from https://www.nice.org.uk/guidance/ng193/chapter/Recommendations#managing-chronic-primary-pain [accessed 31 January 2026].

Osborn, M. and Smith, J.A. (1998). The personal experience of chronic benign lower back pain: An interpretative phenomenological analysis. *British Journal of Health Psychology*, 3, 65–83.

Reber, A.S. (1995). *The Penguin dictionary of psychology* (2nd edition). Penguin.

Rodham, K. (2020). *Self-management for persistent pain: The blame, shame and inflame game?* Palgrave Macmillan.

Scott, W. and McCracken, L.M. (2015). Psychological flexibility, acceptance and commitment therapy, and chronic pain. *Current Opinion in Psychology*, 2, 91–96. https://doi.org/10.1016/j.copsyc.2014.12.013.

Strand, E.B., Varsi, C., Børøsund, E., et al. (2025). Changes in cognitions, coping, pain and emotions after 12-months access to the digital self-management programme EPIO. *Frontiers in Psychology*, 16, 1540852. doi: 10.3389/fpsyg.2025.1540852.

Vaikar, S. and Swaminathan, N. (2026). Exploring factors influencing adherence to home exercise program among patients with chronic musculoskeletal pain: A scoping review. *Physiotherapy Quarterly*, 34(1), 1–6.

Wang, Y., Aaron, R., Attal, N., and Colloca, L. (2025). An update on non-pharmacological interventions for pain relief. *Cell Reports Medicine*, 6, 101940. https://doi.org/10.1016/j.xcrm.2025.101940.

Welsch, P., Petzke, F., Klose, P., and Häuser, W. (2020). Opioids for chronic osteoarthritis pain: An updated systematic review and meta-analysis of efficacy, tolerability and safety in randomized placebo-controlled studies of at least 4 weeks double blind duration. *European Journal of Pain*, 24, 685–703.

7

SO WHAT CAN WE ALL DO TO HELP THOSE WHO LIVE WITH PERSISTENT PAIN LIVE WELL, IN SPITE OF THEIR PERSISTENT PAIN?

INTRODUCTION

In this final chapter, I bring together the different strategies, tools, interventions, and tips that have been shared over the course of this book. Together, we have explored what it is like to live with persistent pain, why explaining pain to another person is so hard, and why it is difficult to manage your own pain. We have also looked at whether laughter and swearing might have an impact on persistent pain as well as thought about what psychology has to offer those with persistent pain.

Given the predictions that, as the population ages, persistent pain will become an even greater issue over the next few decades, living well in spite of persistent pain is becoming ever more important (McGhie and Grady, 2016). With this in mind, the intention behind this chapter is to highlight that there are things that we can all do that will make a positive difference to those who are living with persistent pain. While most of the points I make will be practical, I recognise that there will also be some points that might be described as wishful thinking. These are the things that are outside our immediate

DOI: 10.4324/9781003649854-7

control but that, if put in place, could make a huge difference to the lives of those who live with persistent pain. I will start with a focus on the bigger picture, the 'wishful thinking' elements, before moving on to things that are more within immediate reach.

WISHFUL THINKING

Richard Horton (1995) challenges us to question what we know about disease when he asks us to question what we assume is normal. In doing so, he draws from the work of a French doctor called Canguilhem (pronounced 'Con-Ghee-Em'), born in 1904, who defined health as the ability to adapt to challenges posed by the environment. This is, I think, an important reminder that we should always take the time to find out about a person's wider context when we are exploring how we can better help them to live well with their pain. Some environments are simply too challenging to adapt to when you live with a long-term condition. The environment itself prevents us from living well.

Staying with this idea, Tom Shakespeare (2021, p. 117) wonders how decisions are made about what to prioritise. There are global targets to address hunger, so why not pain. He asks: 'Why is there never a similar target for eliminating pain, or reducing pain?'. He suggests that medication cannot ultimately control pain 'unless you are willing to be comatose'. So, if pain cannot be medicated away, he says, we should still expect our health professionals to have received excellent education in pain medicine, and to recognise and validate the pain we experience. This is an important point about education and training. Heath and Phillip (2020) note that, globally, chronic pain is among the leading causes of years lived with disability, yet primary care practices often lack the support and training to address this huge problem. Similarly, Lusher and Murray (2018) highlight the mismatch between the high prevalence of persistent pain and the low number of hours devoted to teaching medical students about pain. Given that up to half of the UK adult population will experience chronic pain, it is likely that all health professionals will have patients who are living with long-term pain, yet the number of hours of teaching offered is woefully low (Briggs et al., 2015).

Heath and Phillip (2020) go on to suggest that, in addition to the amount of training offered being limited, during that training medical students are exposed to negative attitudes towards people who live with persistent pain. They are also generally taught that if a patient presents with pain, they should prescribe a painkiller. Also, persistent pain can be frustrating for the doctor who has learned in medical school that 'patients have things wrong with them and there's always a medical cause for it and you've got to try and find it' (Howman et al., 2016, p. 7). Better training would avoid health professionals becoming anxious about their inability to fix a person. This reduction in emotion could then allow the health professional to listen properly to what it is that the person living with long-term pain has to say about their experience. Until this training and awareness raising is complete, health professionals will continue to feel frustrated. Furthermore, they often lack support or referral options for people with persistent pain. For example, Jamil and colleagues (2025) note that a standard 10-minute GP appointment is not enough time to develop a collaborative approach to care. So the system itself disempowers both the GP and the patient. The patient is not given enough time to explain their experiences and so does not feel heard, and the GP falls back on medical solutions because of the limited time and their minimal training in pain education.

Other challenges for GPs have been highlighted in a study by Larsen and colleagues (2024). GPs reported having to coordinate the appointments with multiple specialists in a system that was not joined up. They felt that the system drove what they considered an overuse of tests combined with a lack of patient education. They called for a more connected system that brought the different disciplines together. This, of course, brings its own challenges, some of which were explored by Gleadhill and colleagues (2021), who noted that the World Health Organization (WHO) defined integrated care as a continuum of services delivered by a system organised around the health needs of people rather than diseases (WHO, n.d.). Therein lies the problem, for our health system in the United Kingdom is based around diseases. This challenge is described clearly by Heath and Phillip (2020, p. 2):

> Attempting to address the biological process and social needs and psychological components of chronic pain may appear to consume time and invite issues, such as social needs, that providers may feel they are unable to address. Yet, this is precisely why integration is required. The nature of chronic pain means that treatment involves these components and that healthcare professionals operating in silos cannot deliver best-quality, evidence-based care. Treatment of chronic pain needs to be publicly reframed as a condition, like any other, that deserves proactive, evidence-based treatment. Healthcare delivery should be restructured to ensure that healthcare needs of the most vulnerable are met. This is a call to action for practices and providers to strive for excellence, not simply survival, in care for this patient population.

So it is worth remembering here that our health professionals are doing their best within a system that is not designed for chronic conditions. My wishful thinking is the same as that expressed by Heath and Phillip (2020) and the WHO (n.d.). I wish for properly integrated care.

HEALTH PROFESSIONALS

Given the bigger-picture systemic issues I have just outlined, health professionals might be forgiven for feeling overwhelmed. However, there are still things that can be done within the constraints of the current system. Much of what I write about in this section stems from the work of McCaffery (1968), who, you will remember, said that pain was whatever the person experiencing it says it is. This seems to be an easy-to-understand statement but, as we have seen in earlier chapters, the work of De Ruddere and colleagues (2011, 2012, 2013, 2014) has shown that, in order to be taken seriously, patients have to do a lot of work, including being likeable and not looking too healthy (even though we know pain is invisible) in order to be taken seriously (Kool et al., 2009). I will highlight six behaviours that, if consistently adopted by health professionals, could vastly improve the experience of the person living with persistent pain.

(1) Believe the patient

Vase and colleagues (2025) suggest acknowledging that the patient's pain is real and that it is crucial that you, as a health professional, are a supportive ally. They also suggest that the person's core beliefs need to be assessed as part of the data-gathering to inform the creation of a tailored plan to support that person. They propose asking patients to share 'the best explanation that they have ever been given for their pain to assess what is believed, how strongly that belief is held, and how metaphors and language are used in sense-making' (Vase et al., 2025, p. 1787). They also suggest that, if health professionals explored the patient's belief that suffering was an inevitable consequence of chronic pain, they would be likely to be able to identify the patient's underlying fears. After all, saying you cannot do something is a way of protecting yourself from a feared negative outcome rather than being a factual statement.

(2) Work in 'collaborment'

A second thing health professionals can do is to learn to work in collaboration with their patients. This requires health professionals to reframe their view of their role. Rather than sole expert, they could learn to accept that the person in pain is an expert both in their pain and in their own life context. This is often reported as challenging. For example, in the work of Grudniewicz and colleagues (2023) clinicians often endorsed the idea of setting goals with patients, but the goals tended to relate to disease management targets rather than patient priorities. This is important because if the health professionals cannot recognise that the patient is an expert in their own life they will fail to help the person in pain live their best life. Instead, the interventions will be focused on the life the health professional thinks is a most appropriate. Padilha and colleagues (2017) explored this when they designed a study that aimed to support decision-making and encourage information-sharing between professionals and patients who were living with chronic obstructive pulmonary disease. A researcher sat in on clinics and asked the nursing staff questions about what they were doing. The questions were designed to encourage the nurses to reflect on their practice. This began to change the way that nurses worked with their patients. The focus of the nurses moved from the condition to placing the patient at the core of what they did. One patient said: 'Now the nurses respond to my daily life problems. With their help I can do things I'd already given up doing. I know what I can do to avoid getting worse' (Padilha et al., 2017, p. 126). This is a positive example of how a small change in practice can make a difference to the patients.

(3) Communicate accessibly

A third thing health professionals can do is make sure that they communicate in an accessible way. It is important that in conversation, in email, and in paper correspondence, information is shared in a way that is accessible to those with different literacy levels. For example, Nijs and colleagues (2015, p. 217) note that information and awareness raising is vital, and that without it 'patients often misunderstand the neuroscience message and believe that they are being told the pain is all in your head'. They go on to say that an information leaflet or explanatory handbook should also be used. They make it clear, too, that such an approach 'assumes that the patient will be intelligent enough to understand the information provided' (Nijs et al., 2015, p. 217). This is such an important point to highlight. Information written with such assumptions is little more than information written *by experts*. What is needed is information written *for patients*.

Evidence for this need can be found in the statistics from the UK Department for Education (2024) highlighting that 18 per cent of adults in England aged 16 to 65 years are described as having very poor literacy skills. The National Literacy Trust (n.d.) website explains: 'this means they can understand short straightforward texts on familiar topics accurately and independently, and obtain information from everyday sources but reading information from unfamiliar sources or on unfamiliar topics could cause problems. This is also known as being functionally illiterate.'

With almost one in five adults having low literacy levels, it is clear that the assumptions identified by Nijs and colleagues (2015), that patients need to be intelligent enough to understand the information, are prejudiced and unhelpful. After all, if a patient cannot understand the information, they cannot make use of nor learn from that information. Patients should not be made to feel inadequate if they do not understand the information. Sharing information that is difficult to understand makes it harder for patients to ask questions. With this in mind, I used to say to the people I was working with that if ever they did not understand something I said, it would always be because I had not explained it well. In other words, the problem was my ability to explain, not their ability to understand. Indeed, in my opinion, it is the responsibility of the health professionals to ensure that all information is presented, delivered, and taught in a way that is accessible to patients. We should not be placing the burden of making sense of information on our patients. We should instead do the work of translating information so that it is meaningful for whoever we are working with. And then we should double check their understanding. The bottom line is that it should not be difficult to ensure that all information (letters, leaflets, verbal) that is provided to patients should be accessible.

(4) Avoid patient blaming

The fourth thing health professionals can do is avoid patient blaming (see Sullivan & Tripp, 2024). Patient blaming is not a new problem in the management of chronic pain. The clinical literature provides numerous examples of how individuals with chronic pain have been blamed for contributing to their pain condition or for failing to improve following treatment. One way in which patients are blamed can be found in the reports written by health professionals about their patients who are living with long-term health conditions. The language chosen to describe such patients can be stigmatising. This includes the use of disrespectful terms for patients as well as language that firmly places blame on the patients for their health condition. Researchers exploring diabetes, sickle cell disease, and chronic pain have highlighted this as a challenging issue to address (see, for example, the work of Himmelstein et al., 2022; Park et al., 2021; Sedney et al., 2023).

The number and type of terms used to blame people living with pain is extensive. Indeed, Carr (2016) wrote a paper titled 'Patients with Pain Need Less Stigma, Not More'. McArthur and colleagues (2026) note that stigma is not just about a negative way of seeing another person, it can also inform the judgements of other people. If stigmatising language is used in patient notes and other communications, it can impact on how other health professionals view that person. In Chapter 6, I shared the example of Diane who, after finding it impossible to cope with exercise machines, was subsequently labelled 'non-compliant'. This label casts doubt on Diane's willingness to follow health advice and could shape future health professionals' views of her.

Terms identified in a study of stigmatising language in the electronic health record by McArthur and colleagues (2026), included 'difficult patient', 'drug seeking', 'fake', 'in denial', 'malingerer', 'non-compliant', and 'unmotivated'. Since hospital admission notes are read by all staff who will be providing care, the use of stigmatising language can have a far-reaching negative impact by influencing the impressions and attitudes of other health professionals involved in a patient's treatment. It has been suggested that stigmatising language might reflect conscious or unconscious negative biases health professionals hold about specific types of patients or certain types of health conditions. Whatever it signifies, health professionals would do well to become more aware of their language and the power it has, not only on their patients but also on how their colleagues may then approach these patients after having read the descriptions in the notes.

(5) Listen to and hear your patient

When a health professional listens to and hears their patient, it can make an enormous and positive difference to the patient experience. This is clearly shown in the work of Arman & Hök (2016) who wrote of participants' stories of suffering and how transformative it was for them when they felt seen and heard. One participant said: 'The way they received and welcomed me. Their friendliness, their view of the human being. [...] For many years, I think I have lived in a world where I haven't belonged. I appreciate that they see the entire me' (Arman and Hök, 2016, p. 378).

(6) Remember the bigger picture (life context)

It is very important that health professionals remember the bigger picture because our life context impacts on us in many ways. A health professional who does not explore their patients' life contexts cannot understand the impact of their pain and their ability to manage their pain. This is explained well by Stilwell and Harman (2019), who summarise the words of philosopher Evan Thompson (2014):

> Saying that pain is in the brain is like saying flight is in a bird's wings. A brain is needed to have pain and wings are needed to fly – but to understand pain or flight, one needs to consider the whole picture and the relational nature between things like a person (with a body/brain) and their social/environmental context; or the bird in the atmosphere. It follows that the experience of pain will not be found in the blood, brain or other bodily tissues. The tissues in the body or the networks in the brain are not the key to pain – instead they are pieces of a larger system [...]. This always involves the environment that we shape, and that shapes us.
>
> (Stilwell and Harman, 2019, p. 655)

RESEARCHERS

Researchers have an important role to play in ensuring that the work they complete captures the experience of the wider patient population, not just some groups of patients. This might mean researchers rethinking the way in which research is done. McCracken (2023) raises an important point about randomised controlled trials (also known as RCTs). These are considered to be the best way of testing whether a treatment works. I found it gratifying to read this paper because for many years I have been wondering about just how useful RCTs are. I recognise that they are a useful way of testing an idea, but they never seemed to me to be useful for my work as a practising psychologist. The patients who were eligible to take part in RCTs bore very little resemblance to the patients with whom I used to work. In this key paper, McCracken (2023) reports on work that is showing that the results based on group data (the people who take part in RCTs) are different to those that are based on individual data. He argues that we should be focusing more on our patients and watching more closely how their conditions change over time. McCracken says: 'If we intend to personalise pain management, perhaps first and foremost, there is need for a change in mindset.' He argues that we should move towards highly practical treatment delivery guided by application and impact testing of evidence-based methods associated with evidence-based processes of change in the individual case. In other words, with the individual patient's needs in focus and their goals as the measure of success. I could not agree more.

There is also work to be done in the research world in terms of ensuring we set up systems to collect data that allows us to explore the diversity of experience of persistent pain. Leach and colleagues' (2024) paper showed that we are often failing to record the ethnicity of the patients who complete pain management programmes. Without this data we are unable to understand barriers and facilitators that impact on different patient populations and, more importantly, we are unable to design pain services that will remove inequality of access. For an example of why we should pay attention to this, see the work of Bull and colleagues (2023) who explored the experiences of people from diverse ethnic backgrounds and gained insight into the kinds of adaptations that could be made to their group pain programmes that would make a meaningful difference for this population. Along similar lines, Janevic and colleagues (2022, p. 723):

> It is time for the pain research community to adopt practices that reflect a commitment to greater diversity in our studies, and to the promotion of equity in pain care and outcomes. Pain prevalence continues to rise steadily, with causes not fully understood, and minoritized and marginalized groups continue to be disproportionately affected by pain and its effects.

In short, there are two key areas that researchers can focus on that would bring a positive benefit to those who live with persistent pain. First, ensure that research is designed in collaboration with people who live with persistent pain – proper collaboration that fully involves people who live with persistent pain. This will ensure that what is being researched is of interest and of practical use to those who live with persistent pain. Second, researchers should collect pain data that capture the experiences of all parts of the population. As a minimum, data collected should include gender, age, ethnicity, and socioeconomic status. We saw in Chapter 1 just how important these characteristics are. If we know people have different pain experiences because of their gender, their ethnicity, where they live, their financial capital, their literacy levels, then we should be insisting that research explores these things in depth.

PEOPLE WHO DO NOT LIVE WITH PERSISTENT PAIN

Around half of the population will experience persistent pain in their lifetime. This means that around half the population will not have that experience. As we have established, it can be difficult to understand the challenges facing a person who lives with persistent pain. Pain is an internal experience that is very difficult to describe. Whether or not the persistent pain experience of another is understood, there are some things that people who do not live with persistent pain themselves could consider doing, things that would make a positive difference to those who do live with persistent pain.

A common issue identified in the paper written by Nortvedt and colleagues (2016) was the reaction of co-workers and managers. They developed a theme that they labelled 'Rejected at the workplace'. This theme was summarised by Toye and colleagues (2021, p. 5):

> I am rejected at work by managers and coworkers. They don't understand pain. They trivialize my pain. They judge me. They are indifferent. They condemn. Pain and sadness are invisible. I can't explain my pain. They think I can't do a good job. It is humiliating and shameful at work. I am excluded.

This quote pulls together many themes that have been explored in this book. At its centre is the difficulty of seeing, understanding, and believing another person's pain. I quoted Tom Shakespeare (2021) in Chapter 3: he likened hearing about another person's pain being as boring as being invited to look at somebody else's holiday photographs. People cannot see the pain and, over time, they become bored and indifferent. Instead of considering how a person might be helped, people can be sidelined and excluded. As has already been discussed in this book, we have become so used to our health service being able to mend us, that when pain cannot be fixed, it is difficult to understand. And when something is hard to understand, we can become quick to judge. People who live with persistent pain know this. Often, they have experienced this. For example, when writing about their experiences as academics living with chronic illness, Wilkinson and Wilkinson (2023) shared their worries about how colleagues and students might respond to them because of their pain conditions, as well as their fears that their career progression would be impacted. One of the authors described a time when she and her colleague were moving offices. The two of them needed to reach an agreement about the new office layout. However, although the author needed to be able to face the door because her condition made it painful to turn around to see who was coming in, she recalled:

> I did not tell my office buddy the extent of my reasoning, only that I have 'trouble with my neck'. I prefer colleagues to consider my issue as something that is temporary and fleeting and not something that is permanent.

A similar story was shared by a patient with whom I used to work. She chose the name 'Sarah' for the write-up of her experiences. This is an extract from our conversation (Rodham, 2015, p. 57):

Sarah: People have started noticing it [complex regional pain syndrome, CRPS] at work.
Karen: What do they say?
Sarah: They ask me what is wrong. [laughs]
Karen: You are laughing – what do you say?
Sarah: I don't tell them about it. I don't even tell them about the CRPS.
Karen: So they don't know there is anything wrong with you?
Sarah: They do know I have a bad leg, but don't know what is wrong with it. Why have I chosen not to tell them? Because they are going to be the same, I think, [...] will probably turn round and say it is all in my head.

The fears felt and experienced by these people and others who live with persistent pain are commonly shared in the research. Indeed, the series of studies published by De Ruddere and colleagues (2012, 2013, 2014) show that these fears and worries are not unfounded. It is therefore not a surprise that Wilkinson and Wilkinson (2023) gave an example where the long-term nature of their pain was hidden. The effort it takes to hide this and keep it a secret is huge. Imagine if we were able to simply believe someone when they said they were in pain. And then imagine if we were able to explore with that person what we might be able to do that would make their life more manageable. Imagine what they could do with the extra energy and focus they would have when they felt it was safe to share that they live with persistent pain. In short, what people who do not live with persistent pain can do to help reduce the challenges facing those who do live with persistent pain boils down to McCaffery's (1968) statement that pain is whatever the person experiencing it says it is. Unfortunately, we know from the work of Scott and colleagues (2025) that people who show their high level of pain can be judged unfavourably. Perhaps they wince or guard their affected limb. This marks them out as being different and leads to negative judgements being drawn. If people who do not live with persistent pain could learn to question their potentially biased judgements about the person in pain, many challenges facing those who live with persistent pain would reduce. Becoming aware of assumptions and biases held, and then reflecting on them when noticed, can change behaviour.

PEOPLE WHO LIVE WITH PERSISTENT PAIN

Of course, people who live with persistent pain can also do things that will help them to live well, in spite of living with persistent pain. In Chapter 4, I explored the attributes that Van de Velde and colleagues (2019) had identified from their review of the literature. These attributes were solely focused on the role of the individual in managing their own pain. If all ten attributes were to be achieved, an awful lot was being expected of the person living with persistent pain. Without wishing to add to the challenges facing people who are living with persistent pain, it is also important to highlight the things that they can do. For example, Joanne, speaking about the joint responsibility of health professionals and people who live with pain, was quoted in a study by Wilson and colleagues (2017, p. 101). She said: 'They are human (laughs). They are just people that want to help you. And I think that if you are willing to help as well, if you are willing to help yourself, that is half the battle.'

In order to be able to work with health professionals, those who live with persistent pain are faced with the challenge of accepting their new normal. Until some acceptance has been achieved, it will be difficult for such people to move forward with their lives. Acceptance can involve reframing how they see things. It involves letting go of, and grieving for, imagined futures:

> It took me two years to learn to accept it and learn to hold up ... you can't understand ... I had been so healthy and quite suddenly I had all these symptoms. I had to learn to accept ... and then little by little I regained some hope, but it took a long time.
>
> (Wuytack and Miller, 2011, p. 5)

One of the patients I worked with when I practised in the NHS shared her experiences of coming to terms with how her life had changed now that she lived with complex regional pain syndrome. She said:

> But, erm, I've got to try to adapt and think well. This is who I am as well, and my life's just different now. It is no good sitting there and thinking 'I used to get up there and do all that wallpapering' or this, that and the other. I'm not doing that, so I'll have to work out the coping strategies.
>
> (Rodham, 2015, p. 90)

Acceptance also involves imagining and then putting into practice alternative futures. In effect when you are adjusting to life with persistent pain, you are also involved in a process of restructuring how you see yourself. For example, Hållstam and colleagues (2015) quoted a participant who spoke about working to understand how to put cognitive behaviour therapy into practice:

> The penny's dropped. I started to realize that there was a link between my pain and my own thoughts and actions. I could then start to manage things differently. In pain management they gave me a proper explanation of why I have this pain. They acknowledged the reality of my pain and made me feel accepted as an individual.

Accepting the change in life context as well as understanding and making connections between the things that help or get in the way of their ability to cope with the pain, helps people who live with pain to see what they could do, and also *why* they could do these things. Some of this is all about learning to trust the process. Living with persistent pain is difficult, frustrating, challenging. It can be hard to accept that there is work to be done to learn how to live well with persistent pain. Working with supportive health professionals who can encourage the person in pain to 'stick with it' can reap rewards for the person in pain. Emily, quoted in Wilson and colleagues (2017, p. 102) shared her strong reaction to the physiotherapist with whom she was working on the pain management programme she was completing. She said:

> I wanted to punch her between the eyes and run away, but I guess they kind of, everybody on the team are like, 'just stick with it' and you do, and then you realise why you stuck with it ... and then it starts making sense. It's a bit of a relief as well I think.

Toye and colleagues (2021) conclude that the core skill for a person living well in spite of persistent pain is the ability to accept what has happened and, in the light of that acceptance, to reframe their focus. At its most basic, instead of focusing on what is lost, looking with open curiosity about what is possible – in spite of the pain.

FURTHER RESOURCES

Haines, S. (2015). *Pain is really strange*. Singing Dragon.

REFERENCES

Arman, M. and Hök, J. (2016). Self-care follows from compassionate care: Chronic pain patients' experience of integrative rehabilitation. *Scandinavian Journal of Caring Sciences*, 30, 374–381.

Briggs, E.V., Battelli, D., Gordon, D., et al. (2015). Current pain education within undergraduate medical studies across Europe: Advancing the Provision of Pain Education and Learning (APPEAL) study. *BMJ Open*, 5, e006984.

Bull, E., Young, D., Etchebarne, A., and Malpus, Z. (2023). Understanding ethnic minority service user experiences of being invited to and attending group pain management programmes: A qualitative service evaluation. *British Journal of Pain*, 17(1), 58–70.

Carr, D.B. (2016). Patients with pain need less stigma, not more. *Pain Medicine*, 17, 1391–1393.

De Ruddere, L., Goubert, L., Prkachin, K.M., et al. (2011). When you dislike patients, pain is taken less seriously. *Pain*, 152(10), 2342–2347.

De Ruddere, L., Goubert, L., Stevens, M., et al. (2013). Discounting pain in the absence of medical evidence is explained by negative evaluation of the patient. *Pain*, 154(5), 669–676.

De Ruddere, L., Goubert, L., Stevens, M.A.L., et al. (2014). Health care professionals' reactions to patient pain: Impact of knowledge about medical evidence and psychosocial influences. *The Journal of Pain*, 15(3), 262–270.

De Ruddere, L., Goubert, L., Vervoot, T., et al. (2012). We discount the pain of others when pain has no medical explanation. *The Journal of Pain*, 13(12), 1198–1205.

Department for Education, UK (2024). Survey of adult skills 2023 (PIAAC): National Report for England, research report. Department for Education, UK.

Gleadhill, C., Kamper, S.J., Lee, H., and Williams, C.M. (2021). Exploring integrated care for musculoskeletal and chronic health conditions. *Journal of Orthopaedic & Sports Physical Therapy*, 51(6), 264–268.

Grudniewicz, A., Gray, C.S., Boeckxstaens, P., et al. (2023). Operationalizing the chronic care model with goal-oriented care. *Patient Centred Outcomes Research*, 16, 569–578.

Hållstam, A., Löfgren, M., Svensén, C., and Ståalnacke, B.M. (2015). Patients with chronic pain: One-year follow-up of a multimodal rehabilitation programme at a pain clinic. *Scandinavian Journal of Pain*, 10, 36–42.

Heath, L. and Phillip, A. (2020). Chronic pain care: Time for excellence. *Family Medicine and Community Health*, 8, e000285.

Himmelstein, G., Bates, D., and Zhou, L. (2022). Examination of stigmatizing language in the electronic health record. *JAMA Network Open*, 5(1), e2144967.

Horton, R. (1995). George Canguilhem: Philosopher of disease. *Journal of the Royal Society of Medicine*, 88, 316–319.

Howman, M., Walters, K., Rosenthal, J., et al. (2016). 'You kind of want to fix it don't you?': Exploring general practice trainees' experiences of managing patients with medically unexplained symptoms. *BMC Medical Education*, 16, 27. doi: 10.1186/s12909-015-0523-y.

Jamil, S., Page, K., Suleman, A., et al. (2025). Rethinking pain: A paradigm shift in primary care for chronic pain via community-based, culturally responsive GP support. *Pain Management*, 15(12), 1015–1025.

Janevic, M.R., Mathur, V.A., Booker, S.Q., et al. (2022). Making pain research more inclusive: Why and how. *The Journal of Pain*, 23(5), 707–728.

Kool, M., van Middendorp, H., Boeije, H.R., and Geenen, R. (2009). Understanding the lack of understanding: Invalidation from the perspective of the patient with fibromyalgia. *Arthritis and Rheumatism*, 61(12), 1650–1656.

Larsen, J.B., Borregaard, P., Thomsen, J.L., et al. (2024). Improving general practice management of patients with chronic musculoskeletal pain: Interdisciplinarity, coherence and concerns. *Scandinavian Journal of Pain*, 24, 20230070.

Leach, E., Ndosi, M., Jones, G.T., et al. (2024). Access to chronic pain services for adults from minority ethnic groups in the United Kingdom (UK): A scoping review. *Journal of Racial and Ethnic Health Disparities*, 11, 3498–3508.

Lusher, J. M. and Murray, E. (2018). Contested pain: Managing the invisible symptom. *International Journal of Health*, 1, 2. DOI:10.4172/IJGH.1000105.

McArthur, A., Ahmad, A., Links, A.R., et al. (2026). How words discredit: A taxonomy of stigmatising language in the electronic health record. *Patient Education and Counseling*, 147, 109520.

McCaffery, M. (1968). *Nursing practice theories related to cognition, bodily pain, and man-environment interactions*. University of Los Angeles.

McCracken, L.M. (2023). Personalized pain management: Is it time for process-based therapy for particular people with chronic pain? *European Journal of Pain*, 27, 1044–1055.

McGhie, J. and Grady, K. (2016). Where now for UK chronic pain management services? *British Journal of Anaesthesia*, 116, 159–162.

National Literacy Trust (n.d.). https://literacytrust.org.uk/parents-and-families/adult-literacy/ [accessed 13 February 2026].

Nijs, J., Girbés, E.L., Lundberg, M., et al. (2015). Exercise therapy for chronic musculoskeletal pain: Innovation by altering pain memories. *Manual Therapy*, 20, 216–220. https://www.sciencedirect.com/science/article/pii/S1356689X14001301.

Nortvedt, L., Lohne, V., Kumar, B.N., and Hansen, H.P. (2016). A lonely life: A qualitative study of immigrant women on long-term sick leave in Norway. *International Journal of Nursing Studies*, 54, 54–64.

Padilha, J.M., Sousa, P.A.F., and Pereira, F.M.S. (2017). Nursing clinical practice changes to improve self-management in chronic pulmonary obstructive disease. *International Nursing Review*, 65(1), 122–130.

Park, J., Saha, S., Chee, B., et al. (2021). Physician use of stigmatizing language in patient medical records. *JAMA Network Open*, 4(7), e2117052.

Rodham, K. (2015). *Learning to cope with CRPS/RSD: Putting life first and pain second.* Singing Dragon.

Scott, W., Buchman, D.Z., and Vasilou, V.S. (2025). The multi-dimensional stigma of chronic pain: A narrative review. *Current Opinion in Psychology*, 62: 101980.

Sedney, C., Dekeseredy, P., Singh, S.A., and Holbein, M. (2023). Stigmatizing language expressed towards individuals with current or previous OUD who have pain and cancer: A qualitative study. *Journal of Pain and Symptom Management*, 65(60), 553–561.

Shakespeare, T. (2021). 'This is going to hurt me more than it hurts you': The problem of pain. In P. Wemyss-Gorman (ed.), *Innovative approaches to chronic pain: Understanding the experience of pain and suffering and the role of healing*. Jessica Kingsley Publishers.

Stilwell, P. and Harman, K. (2019). An enactive approach to pain: Beyond the biopsychosocial model. *Phenomenology and the Cognitive Sciences*, 18, 637–665.

Sullivan, M.J.L. and Tripp, D.A. (2024). Pain catastrophizing: Controversies, misconceptions and future directions. *The Journal of Pain*, 25(3), 585–587.

Thompson, E. (2014). The embodied mind: An interview with Evan Thompson. https://tricycle.org/magazine/embodied-mind/ [accessed 15 February 2026].

Toye, F., Belton, J., Hannink, E., et al. (2021). A healing journey with chronic pain: A meta-ethnography synthesizing 195 qualitative studies. *Pain Medicine*. doi: 10.1093/pm/pnaa373.

Van de Velde, D., De Zutter, F., Satink, T., et al. (2019). Delineating the concept of self-management in chronic conditions: A concept analysis. *BMJ Open*, 9, e027775. doi: 10.1136/bmjopen-2018-027775.

Vase, L., Wager, T.D., and Eccleston, C. (2025). Opportunities for chronic pain self-management: Core psychological principles and neurobiological underpinnings. *Lancet*, 405, 1781–1790.

Wilkinson, S. and Wilkinson, C. (2023). Pain, no gain? A joint-autoethnography of our working lives as academics with chronic illnesses. *International Journal of Changes in Education*, 1(1), 4–10.

Wilson, S., Chaloner, N., Osborn, M., and Gauntlett-Gilbert, J. (2017). Psychologically informed physiotherapy for chronic pain: Patient experiences of treatment and therapeutic process. *Physiotherapy*, 103, 98–105

WHO, World Health Organization (n.d.). Framework on integrated people-centred health services. https://www.who.int/health-topics/integrated-people-centered-care#tab=tab_1 [accessed 8 February 2026].

Wuytack, F. and Miller, P. (2011). The lived experience of fibromyalgia in female patients: A phenomenological study. *Chiropractic and Manual Therapies*, 19, 22.

FINAL THOUGHTS

Helping people who live with persistent pain to live well in spite of their persistent pain seems to be a very difficult task. The health care system is not set up for people with long-term conditions. It is disjointed and experts often work in splendid isolation. The GP struggles to provide care for many more patients than it is possible to see. The appointments, when you can get them, are short. And yet, in spite of these systemic challenges, there are simple things that can be done that could have a positive impact on a person's pain experience. These simple things are not rocket science. I suppose here, I am referring back to my 'Aha!' moment that I mentioned at the start of this book. That moment when I realised that *mange tout* meant 'eat all' – that the name of the vegetable was telling me how to eat it. I knew *mange* in French meant 'eat' and *tout* meant 'all'. But I did not ever put that learning together. Sherlock Holmes would have shaken his head sadly and said 'You looked but did not see' (or something along those lines).

Patients have said time and again in the research that they simply want to be listened to – and heard. They want to be believed. They want their life context to be understood. They do not want to be dismissed for not engaging with or not prioritising their health. They want to be treated as someone who has expertise in their own condition and their own life context. These are reasonable requests and apply not just to health professionals, but to friends, family, colleagues, employers, and so on. Regardless of the systemic, political, economic, social, and financial challenges, there are things that we can *all* do to help someone to live well, in spite of their persistent pain:

- Listen to what someone is telling you about how they feel.
- Believe them when they tell you about their pain.
- Recognise they are experts in their own experience and their own life context.
- Actively involve them in any decisions (use their expertise).
- Ask them about their life context.
- Be kind.
- Be their ally.

INDEX